APOTHECARY BEAUTY

HEAL, TRANSFORM, AND ACHIEVE LASTING HEALTH AND HAPPINESS

BUNNY MEADOWS

JENNIFER LYNN DEMERS

Table of Contents

Apothecary Beauty

HEAL, TRANSFORM, AND ACHIEVE LASTING HEALTH AND HAPPINESS

INTRODUCTION

Botanical and Mycological remedies have been a cornerstone of health and wellness for centuries, offering natural solutions to the ailments that plague us. For as long as I can remember, I have turned to ancient remedies to heal, restore, and maintain vitality. What began as simple curiosity evolved into a deep passion for herbal wisdom and its transformative power. I am eager to share the knowledge I've gathered, helping others cultivate beauty, health, and self-sufficiency through the timeless art of herbal healing.

A home apothecary is more than just a collection of herbs and remedies; it is your sanctuary of natural healing. By creating your home apothecary, you take control of your health, crafting personalized solutions tailored to your unique needs. A home apothecary offers a path to balance and vitality in a world where stress, pollution, and processed foods have become the norm.

The challenges we face today are numerous. Emotional and physical stress, weakened immune systems, and exposure to harmful chemicals have left many of us feeling depleted and unwell. According to a recent study, over 70% of American adults experience significant stress daily, contributing to a host of health issues. Additionally, the overuse of pharmaceuticals has led to a growing resistance to antibiotics and a reliance on synthetic solutions that often come with unwanted side effects.

"Apothecary Beauty: Heal, Transform, and Achieve Lasting Health and Happiness" is your comprehensive guide to overcoming these challenges through home apothecary's natural and sustainable practices. By harnessing the power of medicinal plants and fungi, you can transform your health, enhance your beauty, and cultivate a deep sense of well-being. This book aims to empower you with the knowledge and skills to create your home apothecary, embracing a holistic approach to health that honors the wisdom of our ancestors while integrating the latest scientific research.

My vision is to reconnect you with the ancestral traditions and natural healing practices lost in the modern world. By embracing the principles of sustainability, self-sufficiency, and ecological responsibility, we can cultivate a new relationship with the earth and the plants that sustain us. By integrating ancient wisdom and modern science, you will discover the tools to achieve lasting health, radiant beauty, and a profound sense of vitality.

The growing interest in natural remedies and self-sufficiency is a testament to the power of this approach. A recent survey found that over 60% of American adults have used complementary or alternative medicine in the past year, with herbal and adaptogen remedies being among the most popular choices. As more people seek natural solutions to their health concerns, the need for accessible and reliable information has never been greater.

Throughout history, cultures around the world have developed their own unique traditions of herbal medicine. From the Ayurvedic practices of India to the Traditional Chinese Medicine of the East, these diverse approaches offer a wealth of knowledge and inspiration for the modern home Apothecarist. Drawing on these global perspectives can create a more holistic and inclusive understanding of natural healing.

In the following pages, you will gain practical skills, scientific knowledge, and the ability to create personalized remedies tailored to your unique health needs. This book offers a comprehensive guide to cultivating your natural pharmacy, from ethical foraging techniques to advanced apothecary methods. You will learn how to identify, grow, harvest, and prepare medicinal plants. Create tinctures, salves, teas, mocktails, and healthy alternatives to everyday items like toothpaste, laundry soap, and shampoo.

I invite you to embark on this journey of exploration and beauty transformation, using the tools and knowledge in this book to foster a more balanced, health-conscious lifestyle. As you delve into the world of home apothecary, you will discover a newfound sense of empowerment and connection to the natural world.

Remember, this book is not just about herbal remedies or adaptogen tonics; it's about cultivating a lifestyle that harmonizes with nature and promotes lasting beauty, health, and happiness. By embracing the wisdom of the past and the potential of the present, you can create a brighter, more vibrant future for yourself and the planet.

Chapter One

Rediscovering Ancient Wisdom

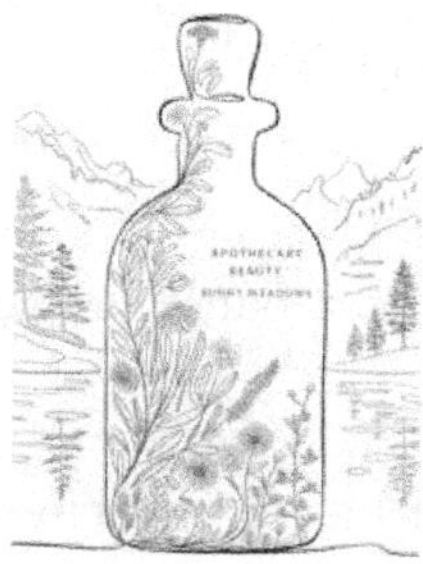

For centuries, herbs have been valued for their beauty, fragrance, and medicinal benefits. Traditional healing systems worldwide, from Traditional Chinese Medicine and Ayurveda to indigenous practices across Africa, the Americas, and Australia, have relied on plant-based remedies to enhance appearance, cognition, relieve discomfort, and restore balance.

There has been a renewed appreciation for these ancient practices as individuals seek to reconnect with nature and incorporate holistic remedies into their daily lives. This revival represents more than a trend. It is a global movement toward sustainable, plant-based healing that blends ancestral wisdom with modern scientific understanding.

Establishing a home apothecary allows individuals to cultivate this tradition within their own spaces, harnessing the power of botanicals for self-care, wellness, and longevity. By learning the foundations of herbal medicine, one can embrace the enduring legacy of plant-based healing while fostering deep connections to the natural world.

Herbalism's roots run deep, entwining with the very foundations of human civilization. It's in Ancient Egypt, health was perceived as a delicate balance between divine forces, with medicinal plants as essential tools in healing and spiritual practice. Egyptian priests who held dual roles as physicians and religious leaders, meticulously employed botanicals. Cumin and fennel are known for their well-documented therapeutic properties and sacred conduits to the gods. These herbs were integral to holistic treatments, reflecting the Egyptians' in-depth understanding of the interconnectedness between medicine, spirituality, and the natural world.

"The Ancient Egyptians prized health, well-being, and personal appearance. Healthiness was next to Godliness, and the priests /physicians, as well as magicians who participated in medical care, viewed health and sickness as a battle between good and evil." Abou El-Soud, Neveen [Source 1].

This reverence for plant-based medicine is documented in surviving medical and magical papyri, including the Ebers Papyrus, Kahun Papyrus, Ramesseum Papyrus, and the Demotic Magical Papyrus, which offer a window into Egyptian medical practices, blending magic and science. The Kahun Gynaecological Papyrus, 1800 BCE, is Egypt's oldest known medical text. It focuses on women's health, such as gynecological diseases, fertility, pregnancy, and contraception. The Ramesseum Papyrus concentrates on eyes, muscles, tendons, pediatrics, and gynecology. The Ebers Papyrus, from around 1550 BC, highlights many topics, including dermatology, dentistry, digestive diseases, migraines, traumatic diseases, and gynecological conditions. The Carlsberg Papyrus VIII covers diseases of the eye and provides much more detail on pregnancy. Focusing mainly on snakebites, the Brooklyn Papyrus speaks of remedial methods for poisons from snakes, scorpions, and tarantulas.

Ancient Egyptian medical papyri contain numerous remedies and recipes focused on vitality, longevity, and overall well-being. The workers who built the pyramids were given garlic and onions to maintain strength and stamina. The Egyptians valued fenugreek for its ability to enhance endurance and promote youthful skin. Special bath infusions of lotus, myrrh, and cedar oil were believed to rejuvenate the body and soul.

Egyptian Vitality Elixir

A Rejuvenating Tonic Inspired by Ancient Egyptian Remedies

Ingredients:

½ cup dried lotus petals or rose petals (sacred in Egyptian culture, promotes relaxation and renewal)

¼ tsp Epsom salt or Dead Sea salt (detoxifying, relieves fatigue)

1 tbsp raw honey (softens skin, antimicrobial)

5-7 drops of essential oils:

Frankincense (enhances vitality, spiritual clarity)

Myrrh (deep healing, strengthens immune function)

Cinnamon or Cardamom (stimulates circulation, warming)

1 tbsp fresh aloe vera gel (moisturizes, soothes skin)

½ cup warm milk (optional) (historically used by Egyptian royalty for glowing skin)

Instructions:

Mix warm water or herbal tea with honey, fenugreek, and cinnamon in a small cup until well blended.

Add the aloe vera gel and stir gently.

If using, add a few drops of food-grade frankincense extract for its ancient medicinal properties.

Sweeten with date juice or syrup, and mix well.

Drink in the morning or before a ritual for enhanced energy and vitality.

Benefits:

✔ *Boosts stamina & energy*

✔ *Supports digestion & detoxification*

✔ *Enhances circulation & mental clarity*

✔ *Balances hormones & vitality*

Ayurveda (the study of life) flourished across the Indian subcontinent as one of the world's oldest medical systems and remains one of India's traditional healthcare systems. Ayurvedic practitioners developed intricate methods to diagnose and treat various ailments, using a holistic approach encompassing diet, lifestyle, and herbal remedies, including oils and common spices. Ayurvedic treatment is unique for each person but begins with internal cleansing (purification). Followed by a special diet of medicines, massage therapy with different oils, yoga, and meditation. Ayurvedic preparations have been found to reduce pain and increase function in people with osteoarthritis. Turmeric, a golden gem of Ayurveda, has been cherished for centuries for its potent anti-inflammatory benefits. From soothing aching joints to promoting radiant skin, this vibrant spice is a powerful example of how ancient wisdom continues to shape modern wellness.

Always consult a qualified Ayurvedic practitioner before starting any new treatment, especially if you have existing medical conditions or are taking medications. Ensure the herbs you purchase are from a reputable source to guarantee purity and potency.

Ayurveda is rich with ancient herbal preparations and recipes specifically designed to enhance vitality, strength, and longevity.

Ayurvedic Vitality Elixir

A Rejuvenating Tonic Inspired by Ancient Ayurvedic Amla

Ingredients:

1 tsp organic Amla powder/ Indian Gooseberry powder (rich in vitamin C and antioxidants, which help strengthen your immune system, protect against infections, and combat oxidative stress). Regular consumption of Amla supports collagen production, promoting glowing skin, stronger hair follicles, and overall cellular rejuvenation.

1 tsp raw, organic honey

½ tsp organic ghee or coconut oil (nourishes tissues deeply, balances hormones, and provides sustained energy throughout the day)

1 cup warm almond milk or coconut milk

Pinch of ground cardamom (improves digestion, alleviates bloating, and enhances gut health)

Pinch of saffron threads (gently uplifts mood, helping reduce stress and anxiety, and enhancing mental clarity and focus)

Dried calendula petals or edible flower petals (optional garnish)

Instructions:

Blend the Amla powder, honey, and ghee (or coconut oil) in a small bowl until it forms a smooth paste.

Warm almond or coconut milk gently in a saucepan over medium-low heat.

Stir the Amla-honey-ghee mixture into the warm milk until fully dissolved.

Add cardamom and saffron threads, stirring gently to release their aromatic qualities.

Simmer the mixture gently for 2–3 minutes to enhance flavors.

Remove from heat and let cool slightly.

Pour into a comforting mug.

Garnish with calendula petals or edible flowers for an elegant, restorative presentation.

Benefits:

✔ *Nourishes tissues deeply*

- ✔ *Provides lasting energy throughout the day*
- ✔ *Enhances mood & mental clarity*
- ✔ *Balances hormones & vitality*

Traditional Chinese Medicine (TCM) is deeply rooted in the belief that humans are a microcosm of the larger universe, where the body, mind, and environment are interconnected. Ancient practitioners observed that well-being is intricately tied to natural rhythms, including the changing seasons, emotional states, and external environmental factors. Just as nature undergoes growth, rest, and renewal cycles, so must the human body maintain balance to thrive.

This holistic perspective led to the development of therapies that addressed physical ailments, lifestyle, emotional health, and environmental influences. TCM recognized that stress, seasonal shifts, diet, and even moon phases could impact health. As a result, its treatments sought to harmonize the body with its surroundings, integrating practices such as seasonal dietary adjustments, meditation, and energy-balancing techniques to maintain equilibrium.

At the heart of TCM is preventive care, a principle that sets it apart from many other traditional healing systems. Unlike reactive medicine, which treats illness once it appears, TCM practitioners aim to identify and correct imbalances before they develop into disease. In fact, ancient Chinese physicians were often compensated based on their ability to keep their patients healthy rather than for treating illness—aligning with the wisdom of the proverb, "Fix the roof while the weather is fair."

This proactive approach resonates strongly with modern wellness trends that emphasize nutrition, stress management, and regular movement to prevent chronic disease. TCM's emphasis on maintaining wellness rather than merely curing illness mirrors contemporary preventive medicine, reinforcing the age-old adage, "An ounce of prevention is worth a pound of cure." By recognizing the interplay between mind, body, and nature, TCM continues to offer valuable insights into achieving long-term health and well-being.

TCM Vitality Elixir

A Rejuvenating Elixir Inspired by Traditional Chinese Medicine

Ingredients:

Ginseng (Ren Shen) – 2 teaspoons dried root or powder (invigorates vital energy, strengthens immunity)

Astragalus (Huang Qi) – 1 tablespoon dried root slices (boosts Qi, strengthens the immune system)

Goji Berries (Gou Qi Zi) – 2 tablespoons dried (enriches Yin, boosts vitality, supports vision)

Longan Fruit (Long Yan Rou) – 1 tablespoon dried fruit (nourishes blood, calms the spirit)

Fresh Ginger – 1-inch piece, sliced (improves digestion)

Cinnamon Stick (Rou Gui) – 1 small stick (warms kidney Yang, enhances circulation)

Raw Honey or Maple Syrup – to taste (optional)

Fresh Lemon Slices – for garnish and added freshness (optional)

Spring or Filtered Water – 4 cups

Instructions:

Rinse goji berries and longan fruit lightly. Combine ginseng, astragalus, goji berries, longan fruit, ginger slices, and cinnamon sticks in a medium saucepan.

Add water and bring to a gentle boil. Immediately reduce the heat and simmer on low, covered, for about 20–30 minutes.

Strain the decoction into a glass container or mason jar.

Cool slightly, then stir in raw honey or maple syrup to taste.

Pour into a favorite cup and garnish with fresh lemon slices if desired. Drink warm or chilled.

Consume once daily as a morning tonic or mid-afternoon rejuvenation.

Benefits:

- ✔ *Boosts immunity & resilience*
- ✔ *Rejuvenates vital energy*
- ✔ *Nourishes Qi and enriches Yin*
- ✔ *Supports vision & boosts vitality*

Meanwhile, in the misty landscapes of ancient Celtic regions, druidic herbalism was shrouded in mystery. Celtic cultures have a rich tradition of herbal medicine, passed down through oral teachings, folklore, and Druidic practices. These traditions emphasized the healing power of plants, their spiritual significance, and their connection to the land.

Celts used plants like mistletoe and foxglove, often in rituals that intertwined magic with medicine. The Celts believed certain trees and herbs held magical and medicinal properties. Oak, holly, and rowan were especially revered. Though much of their knowledge was orally transmitted and thus lost to history, remnants of Celtic herbal practices survive in medieval manuscripts such as the "Meddygon Myddfai." These texts reveal a rich tapestry of plant-based remedies, illustrating how the Celts, like their contemporaries, harnessed the healing power of nature [Source 3]. Celtic tradition, passed down through generations, inspires modern herbalists to honor nature's wisdom.

Herbs were often collected ritually, mindful of lunar cycles, seasons, and natural rhythms, making their herbal remedies holistic practices as well as medicinal preparations. Although precise recipes often weren't documented, oral traditions, herbal lore, and folklore have preserved various ingredients and practices that were believed to boost vitality.

Celtic Vitality Elixir

A Rejuvenating Elixir Inspired by Celtic Tradition

Ingredients:

2 tbsp dried nettle leaves (supports immune function and energy levels and reduces inflammation, allergies, and fatigue)

2 tbsp dried elderflowers (boosts the immune system and soothes respiratory issues, provides gentle stress relief and overall well-being)

1 tbsp dried hawthorn berries (supports circulation and cardiovascular health, reduces inflammation and oxidative stress)

1 tbsp dried rose hips (supports immunity, collagen production, skin health, and vitality)

1 tbsp dried meadowsweet (historically used to ease pain and fever naturally, supporting overall health, digestion, and calming of the nervous system)

Zest and juice of 1 organic lemon

½ cup raw, local honey

2 cups filtered water

Instructions:

Bring water to a gentle simmer; remove from heat.

Add herbs. Cover and steep for 20–25 minutes.

Strain infusion. Stir in lemon zest, juice, and honey.

Bottle in amber-colored glass bottles; refrigerate for up to 3 weeks.

1-2 tbsp daily or add to drinks/ smoothies.

Benefits:

- ✔ *Boosts stamina & energy*
- ✔ *Provides stress relief & reduces inflammation*
- ✔ *Soothes respiratory issues & allergies*
- ✔ *Supports heart health & boosts vitality*

The continuity of these ancient practices is remarkable. During the medieval era, apothecaries became the custodians of herbal wisdom in Europe. They meticulously crafted remedies using age-old recipes, adapting them to discoveries and challenges. This tradition of innovation and preservation continues today as we integrate ancient herbal knowledge with scientific advancements. Modern studies confirm the efficacy of numerous traditional remedies, such as the anti-inflammatory effects of willow bark, a precursor to aspirin. This confluence of old and new strengthens the credibility of herbalism and enriches our understanding of its potential.

In embracing the heritage of herbalism, it is crucial to honor the cultural origins of these practices. Indigenous contributions are often overlooked, yet have shaped the landscape of natural medicine. By acknowledging and respecting these diverse sources, we cultivate an inclusive approach that celebrates the richness of human experience. This holistic perspective enhances our connection to the earth and empowers us to heal ourselves and our communities. It fosters a sense of respect and appreciation for the diverse cultures that have contributed to the field of herbalism, enriching our understanding and practice of it.

Herbalism in Modern Health

Gradually, there's been a noticeable shift back towards the natural world as people increasingly seek alternatives to the often impersonal and chemical-laden solutions of conventional medicine. This resurgence in interest in natural remedies stems from growing concerns about the side effects of pharmaceuticals. Many individuals have experienced adverse reactions or found these medications ineffective, leading them to explore the gentler, more holistic approach that herbalism offers. Coupled with this is the rise of holistic health movements, where wellness is viewed not just as the absence of illness but as a state of balanced well-being encompassing the mind, body, and spirit. The appeal lies in the promise of a healthier lifestyle harmonizing with nature and respects respecting the body's innate ability to heal itself.

Integrating herbalism into modern health practices brings numerous benefits. Herbs can serve as vital supplements, particularly for stress relief. For example, adaptogens like ashwagandha and rhodiola are known for their ability to help the body resist stressors, offering a natural way to manage anxiety and fatigue. Herbal alternatives also provide solutions for common ailments. Chamomile can soothe digestive complaints, while peppermint is known for its effectiveness against headaches.

Peppermint Headache Relief Elixir

A Herbal Peppermint Elixir Ideal for Easing Headaches Naturally

Ingredients:

2 tbsp dried peppermint leaves (or 4 tbsp fresh)

1 tbsp dried lemon balm leaves (optional, calming addition)

1 tbsp dried chamomile flowers (for soothing tension)

1 tsp dried lavender buds (relaxes nerves)

2 cups boiling water

1 tbsp raw honey

Juice from half a fresh lemon (optional)

Instructions:

Steep the herbs. Place peppermint, lemon balm, chamomile, and lavender in a heat-proof container. Pour boiling water over herbs, cover, and let steep for 10–15 minutes.

Strain the herbs through a fine-mesh sieve or cheesecloth into a favorite mug. Add raw honey and stir gently to dissolve.

Stir in lemon juice to brighten the flavor and enhance effectiveness.

To Use:

Sip slowly while warm, inhaling deeply. Peppermint, through its cooling effect and aromatic properties, helps relieve tension headaches.

For added headache relief, gently massage peppermint essential oil diluted in carrier oil on the temples or neck.

Benefits:

- ✔ *Peppermint: Provides a cooling sensation, eases tension and sinus pressure, and alleviates headaches.*
- ✔ *Chamomile & Lavender: Calmingly reduces stress-induced tension.*
- ✔ *Lemon Balm: Relaxing, supports mental clarity, and relieves tension.*

Furthermore, herbs bolster immune system health. Echinacea and elderberry, for instance, fortify the body's defenses, helping to ward off colds and flu. In these ways, herbalism complements conventional wellness routines, offering a well-rounded approach to health management.

Elderberry Immunity Boosting Elixir

A Herbal Elderberry Elixir Ideal for Boosting Immunity

Ingredients:

½ cup dried elderberries (rich in antioxidants)

2 tbsp dried rose hips (high in vitamin C)

1 tbsp dried echinacea root or leaves (immune stimulant)

1 cinnamon stick (warming and antiviral)

3 whole cloves (antimicrobial)

2-inch fresh ginger, sliced (anti-inflammatory)

3 cups filtered water

½ cup raw honey (antibacterial, soothing)

Optional additions:

Juice of 1 fresh lemon

1 teaspoon astragalus root (immune-supporting adaptogen)

Instructions:

Simmer Herbs. Combine elderberries, rose hips, echinacea, cinnamon, cloves, ginger, and water in a saucepan. Bring to a gentle boil, then reduce the heat and simmer uncovered for 30–40 minutes until reduced by about half.

Strain the mixture thoroughly, pressing the herbs to extract all nutrients. Allow the liquid to cool slightly, then stir in raw honey until fully dissolved. Optional lemon juice can be added for added vitamin C and flavor.

Transfer to a clean, sterilized glass bottle or jar. Store refrigerated for up to 2 months.

To Use:

Adults: 1 tablespoon daily for immune support; increase to 2–3 tablespoons daily during illness or stress.

Children (over age 1): 1 teaspoon daily; increase to 2 teaspoons during illness.

Benefits:

- ✔ *Elderberry and Rose hips: Packed with antioxidants and vitamin C to strengthen the immune system.*
- ✔ *Echinacea and Astragalus: Support immune response and enhance resilience to illnesses.*
- ✔ *Ginger, Cinnamon, and Cloves: Anti-inflammatory, antiviral, and warming to stimulate healthy circulation and immune function.*

~

Despite the growing popularity of herbal remedies, misconceptions persist about their efficacy. However, a wealth of research supports using herbs to treat various conditions. Clinical studies have demonstrated the effectiveness of turmeric in reducing inflammation, comparable to some anti-inflammatory drugs but without the associated risks. Health practitioners who incorporate herbal medicine into their practices often report positive outcomes, noting the benefits of these treatments in both acute and chronic cases. These testimonials, coupled with empirical evidence, help dispel doubts and reinforce the legitimacy of herbalism as a viable option for health care.

~

Turmeric Anti-Inflammatory Elixir

A Herbal Turmeric Elixir Ideal for Reducing Inflammation

Ingredients:

1 ½ cups coconut milk or almond milk (anti-inflammatory fats)

1 teaspoon turmeric powder (a potent anti-inflammatory)

½ teaspoon cinnamon powder (anti-inflammatory, antioxidant)

¼ teaspoon freshly ground black pepper (enhances turmeric absorption)

½ teaspoon ground ginger or one teaspoon fresh ginger, grated (anti-inflammatory, supports digestion)

½ teaspoon raw honey or pure maple syrup (optional, to taste)

Optional additions:

½ teaspoon ashwagandha powder (adaptogenic, stress-relieving)

1 teaspoon coconut oil (increases nutrient absorption)

Instructions:

Gently warm the coconut or almond milk over medium-low heat in a saucepan.

Whisk in turmeric, cinnamon, ginger, black pepper, and optional ashwagandha powder. Simmer gently for 5 minutes to blend flavors and enhance absorption.

Remove from heat. Stir in coconut oil (optional, recommended) and sweeten with raw honey or maple syrup to taste.

Pour into a mug and savor slowly while warm.

To Use:

Enjoy 1–2 cups daily, ideally before bed or first thing in the morning, for optimal inflammation reduction.

Benefits:

✔ *Turmeric (Curcumin): Powerful anti-inflammatory and antioxidant.*

✔ *Black Pepper: Enhances turmeric's bioavailability and effectiveness.*

✔ *Cinnamon & Ginger: Anti-inflammatory and digestive support.*

✔ *Ashwagandha: Reduces stress and cortisol-related inflammation.*

Herbalism also represents an accessible and sustainable approach to health, democratizing care in a way that is both cost-effective and eco-friendly. Unlike expensive medications, herbs can often be grown at home, reducing costs and ensuring a fresh supply. This accessibility allows individuals to take charge of their health, cultivating a sense of self-reliance and empowerment. The environmental impact is also minimized; growing herbs requires fewer resources than pharmaceutical production, reducing the carbon footprint and supporting biodiversity. By embracing herbalism, individuals contribute to a more sustainable future, promoting ecological balance while nurturing their well-being.

The growing interest in herbalism reflects a broader desire to reconnect with natural remedies and achieve self-sufficiency. As more individuals turn to this ancient practice, they find relief from ailments, a deeper connection to the earth, and a more mindful approach to living. This trend is supported by recent studies, which indicate a significant increase in the use of complementary medicine, with herbal remedies leading the charge. By integrating these practices into everyday routines, people are rediscovering the power of plants, unlocking their potential to heal and transform lives. Herbalism is a forward-thinking approach that aligns with the contemporary values of sustainability and holistic well-being.

Overcoming the Fear of Misidentification

The task of identifying plants can initially appear overwhelming. The apprehension of mistakenly identifying a plant, given the health implications involved, is both common and justified among beginners. Acknowledging that this fear is a natural step in the learning curve can significantly ease the associated stress. It's essential to understand that expertise in plant identification is cultivated gradually and enriched by persistent exposure and education.

Adopting practical strategies can provide reassurance and clarity for those keen to enhance their identification skills. An effective approach includes leveraging field guides that offer comprehensive images and descriptions, facilitating the differentiation between closely related species. Additionally, mobile applications that utilize advanced technology are indispensable tools. These apps enable users to snap photos of plants and quickly receive information on possible identifications.

Participating in workshops focused on plant identification also proves immensely valuable. These interactive sessions provide direct experience under the tutelage of experienced herbalists, creating a supportive environment for inquiry and learning from mistakes. Turning to credible sources is critical for honing accurate plant identification abilities.

Dandelion Detox and Hormonal Balance Cold Brew

A Herbal Dandelion Cold Brew Ideal for Detox and Hormonal Balance

Ingredients:

1 tbsp Dandelion root (supports liver detox for hormone balance)

1 tbsp Nettle leaf (replenishes iron and vital minerals)

1 tbsp Spearmint (helps regulate estrogen levels)

1 tbsp Lemon Balm (supports stress-related hormone fluctuations)

1 quart Filtered filtered water

Instructions:

Add the fresh, clean herbs to a glass jar.

Fill it with filtered water and let it infuse overnight in the fridge.

Strain and drink throughout the week.

To Use:

Enjoy one cup daily, ideally first thing in the morning, for a gentle detoxing herbal water infusion that will keep your hormones balanced.

Esteemed herbalists have authored books that are a rich source of proven knowledge, while authoritative websites and databases offer current information. Enrolling in online courses led by field experts can further solidify one's understanding and boost confidence. These resources are vital as they lay a solid groundwork of knowledge, enabling learners to sift through and disregard misinformation. Gleaning insights from those who have previously navigated this path can make the journey less intimidating.

Ultimately, mastering plant identification becomes an enriching component of your apothecary practice. The confidence developed through diligent study and practice broadens your herbal knowledge and deepens your bond with the natural world. As you traverse gardens and wild spaces, plants feel like familiar companions, each with its own narrative and value. Recognizing that this fear is a normal part of the learning process can alleviate much of the anxiety. It's crucial to remember that expertise is built gradually through repeated exposure and learning.

Spearmint Brain Health Cold Brew Infusion

A Herbal Spearmint Cold Brew Infusion Ideal for Brain Health

Ingredients:

1 tbsp Gotu kola – improves mental clarity

1 tbsp Ginkgo biloba – enhances cognitive function

1 tbsp Spearmint – supports neurotransmitter health

1 tbsp Dried blueberries – high in brain-protective antioxidants

1 quart Filtered filtered water

Instructions:

Add herbs and berries to a glass jar.

Fill with filtered water and let it infuse overnight in the fridge.

Strain and enjoy throughout the day.

To Use:

A refreshing, slow-infused herbal water to drink throughout the day.

Building proficiency in plant identification is akin to learning a new language. Initially, the vocabulary seems overwhelming, the nuances elusive. But with each new word, each new plant, your fluency grows. There will be moments of doubt, where the fear of getting it wrong resurfaces. Yet, you learn the most through these moments, sharpening your skills with every observation and correction. As you progress, you will find that what once seemed a tangled mass of green becomes an intricate tapestry, rich with diversity and possibility.

In time, the once-daunting task of plant identification becomes a rewarding part of your apothecary practice. The confidence gained through careful study and practice enhances your herbal knowledge and enriches your connection to the natural world. As you walk through gardens and forests, the plants greet you like old friends, each with a story and purpose. This deepened relationship with nature is one of the many rewards of overcoming the fear of misidentification. It reminds us that learning is a lifelong, continually evolving and growing process.

Essential Tools for Apothecaries

Creating a home apothecary requires a thoughtful assembly of tools, each serving a distinct purpose in preparing and storing herbal remedies. Among the most indispensable is the mortar and pestle, a timeless duo used to grind herbs into fine powders or pastes. This tool, often made from granite, marble, or ceramic, provides a tactile connection to the herbs, allowing you to release their essential oils and active compounds. The rhythmic motion of grinding breaks down the plant material and fosters a deeper appreciation for the natural ingredients you are working with. Choosing a high-quality mortar and pestle ensures durability and effectiveness, making every preparation a rewarding experience.

Handmade Healing Salve (Mortar & Pestle Method)

This herbal-infused salve is perfect for wound healing, skin repair, inflammation, burns, cuts, and minor infections. It is made by grinding fresh or dried herbs with a mortar and pestle, releasing their medicinal properties before infusing them into an oil base.

Ingredients:

Healing Herbs (Choose 2–3 or mix all for extra potency)

2 tbsp Dried Calendula Flowers (speeds up wound healing and soothes skin)

2 tbsp Dried Plantain Leaves (helps with cuts, burns, and bug bites)

2 tbsp Dried Comfrey Leaves (supports skin regeneration, but avoid using on deep wounds)

2 tbsp Dried Lavender Buds (antimicrobial, calms skin irritation)

2 tbsp Fresh or Dried Rosemary (fights infections, promotes healing)

Base Ingredients:

½ cup Olive Oil, Coconut Oil, or Jojoba Oil – nourishes and hydrates the skin

1 tbsp Beeswax (or Candelilla Wax for a vegan option) – thickens the salve

5–10 drops Tea Tree or Lavender Essential Oil – adds extra antimicrobial protection

Instructions:

Step 1: Grind the Herbs in the mortar and pestle

Add dried herbs to the mortar.

Using the pestle, grind them into a fine powder or paste.

This helps release their natural oils and medicinal compounds.

Why use a mortar and pestle? Grinding herbs activates their healing properties better than a blender or pre-ground powder.

Complementing the mortar and pestle are glass jars and bottles, which are crucial for storing your herbal creations. These containers, available in various sizes, serve as the guardians of your remedies, preserving their potency and freshness. Opt for amber or cobalt blue glass to shield the contents from harmful UV rays, which can degrade the delicate compounds within. Lids should fit securely, preventing air and moisture from compromising the integrity of your preparations. Whether storing tinctures, infused oils, or dried herbs, these jars and bottles provide a practical and aesthetically pleasing solution, lining your shelves like a vibrant apothecary display.

Modern Chyawanprash Herbal Jam

A Herbal Amla Jam Ideal for Collagen Production

Ingredients:

½ cup organic Amla powder (Indian Gooseberry)

2 tbsp Ashwagandha powder

1 tbsp Shatavari powder

1 tbsp Brahmi powder

½ tsp ground cinnamon

½ tsp ground ginger

¼ tsp ground cardamom

¼ tsp ground cloves

¼ tsp black pepper

½ cup raw honey

¼ cup organic ghee or coconut oil (vegan alternative)

Instructions:

In a mixing bowl, combine all dry herbal ingredients and spices.

Gently melt ghee or coconut oil over low heat.

Remove from heat, allow to cool slightly, then blend into the herbal mixture.

Add raw honey, mixing thoroughly until smooth and well-integrated.

Transfer to a sterilized amber or blue glass jar.

Use: Consume one teaspoon daily on an empty stomach, preferably in the morning, for optimal benefits.

Storage: Store in a cool, dark place or refrigerator for freshness.

Benefits:

- ✔ *Boosts immune health and vitality*
- ✔ *Promotes glowing skin and stronger hair follicles*
- ✔ *Rich in antioxidants and adaptogens*
- ✔ *Supports digestion, mental clarity, and overall cellular rejuvenation*

Strainers and cheesecloth are essential in separating plant material from liquid preparations, ensuring clarity and purity in your final product. Strainers, often crafted from stainless steel, are ideal for larger particles, while cheesecloth, a loosely woven cotton fabric, excels at filtering finer residues. Together, they work to refine your herbal concoctions, leaving you with a clear, smooth liquid ready for use. Investing in high-quality strainers and cheesecloth enhances the quality of your remedies and streamlines the preparation process, making it more efficient and enjoyable.

Royal Egyptian Skin Rejuvenation Bath Infusion

A sacred, rejuvenating bath infusion inspired by the healing rituals of Ancient Egypt.

Ingredients:

½ cup dried lotus petals or rose petals (sacred in Egyptian culture, promotes relaxation and renewal)

¼ cup Epsom salt or Dead Sea salt (detoxifying, relieves fatigue)

1 tbsp raw honey (softens skin, antimicrobial)

5-7 drops of essential oils:

Frankincense (enhances vitality and spiritual clarity)

Myrrh (deep healing, strengthens immune function)

Cinnamon or Cardamom (stimulates circulation, warming)

1 tbsp fresh aloe vera gel (moisturizes and soothes skin)

½ cup warm milk (optional) (historically used by Egyptian royalty for glowing skin)

Instructions:

Prepare an Herbal Infusion:

In a bowl, steep the lotus or rose petals in 2 cups of hot water for 15 minutes.

Strain and set aside the infused liquid.

Prepare the Bath:

Fill the bathtub with warm water.

Stir in Epsom/Dead Sea salt, honey, and essential oils.

Add the aloe vera gel and infused floral water.

For extra luxury, pour in warm milk for a Cleopatra-inspired touch.

Set the Atmosphere:

Light candles or burn myrrh or sandalwood incense.

Play soothing music or a gentle Egyptian harp melody.

Recite an affirmation:

"As the waters cleanse and restore, I awaken my vitality and strength."

Soak for 20-30 minutes, allowing the infusion to work its magic.

Benefits:

- ✔ *Replenishes energy & vitality*
- ✔ *Softens & hydrates skin*
- ✔ *Enhances circulation & relaxation*
- ✔ *Connects to ancient wisdom & ritual self-care*

The materials used in these tools are as important as the tools themselves. Non-reactive containers, such as those made from glass or stainless steel, prevent unwanted chemical interactions that could alter the efficacy of your remedies. Organic and sustainable materials, like natural cotton, cheesecloth and ethically sourced wood for mortar handles, further align your practices with environmental commitment. By choosing quality materials, you ensure that your preparations remain true to their natural origins, unmarred by external contaminants.

When it comes to sourcing these tools, several avenues offer reliable options. Reputable online stores provide a wide selection, allowing you to compare products and read reviews before purchasing. Websites dedicated to herbalism and natural living often feature curated collections of high-quality apothecary tools. Alternatively, local craft and health stores can offer a more tactile shopping experience, where you can assess the weight and feel of a mortar and pestle or inspect the craftsmanship of glass jars firsthand. Building a relationship with local vendors can also provide a sense of community and support.

All-Natural Apothecary Tool Cleaner

A gentle yet effective solution to maintain and purify home apothecary tools naturally.

Ingredients:

1 cup distilled white vinegar (natural disinfectant)

½ cup distilled water (prevents mineral deposits)

1 tbsp witch hazel (gentle antiseptic)

10 drops tea tree essential oil (antibacterial, antifungal)

10 drops lavender essential oil (soothing, antimicrobial)

Optional: 5 drops of lemon or eucalyptus essential oil (extra cleansing and refreshing scent)

Instructions:

Combine vinegar, distilled water, and witch hazel in a glass spray bottle.

Add essential oils, then gently shake to mix thoroughly.

Label the spray bottle clearly for easy use.

Usage:

Spray generously onto tools (spoons, jars, bowls, droppers).

Allow to sit for 2-3 minutes.

Wipe clean thoroughly with a soft cloth or rinse with warm water.

Allow tools to air-dry completely before storage.

Benefits:

✔ *Naturally disinfects without harsh chemicals*

✔ *Safely cleans delicate tools*

✔ *Maintains purity of apothecary ingredients*

✔ *Leaves behind a calming, refreshing aroma*

~

Maintaining your apothecary tools is paramount to their longevity and functionality. Regular cleaning and sterilizing prevent cross-contamination and preserve the purity of each preparation. Mortar and pestle sets should be washed with warm, soapy water and thoroughly dried to avoid moisture buildup. Glass jars and bottles benefit from periodic sterilization, which can be achieved by boiling them in water or using a dedicated sterilizing solution. Strainers and cheesecloth should be rinsed immediately after use, with cheesecloth replaced regularly to maintain effectiveness.

Proper storage techniques further ensure the longevity of your tools. Keep your mortar and pestle in a dry, cool area, away from direct sunlight, which can cause cracking or discoloration. Glass jars and bottles should be stored in a cabinet or pantry, organized by size and function, for easy access. Strainers can be hung to dry, while cheesecloth should be kept in a sealed container to prevent dust accumulation. By caring for your tools, you extend their lifespan and enhance the overall apothecary experience, allowing you to focus on the creative and therapeutic aspects of herbalism.

Ethical Foraging and Sourcing

In the tapestry of herbalism, ethical foraging is a vital thread, weaving together respect for nature with mindful practice. As we explore the natural world, we must approach it with reverence and responsibility, ensuring that our actions are responsible and support, rather than deplete, the ecosystems we cherish. Ethical foraging is not merely a practice; it is a philosophy rooted in the understanding that every plant and every habitat plays a unique role in the web of life. By prioritizing environmental conservation, we protect this delicate balance, ensuring that biodiversity thrives for future generations.

One of the primary tenets of ethical foraging is the protection of biodiversity. When we forage, we must be mindful of the species we harvest, ensuring we do not disrupt the natural balance. Overharvesting can lead to the decline of specific plant populations, affecting the broader ecosystem. By taking only what we need and leaving the rest to flourish, we allow nature to replenish itself. This practice not only preserves the beauty and diversity of our landscapes but also ensures that future foragers can enjoy the same bounty we do today.

As stewards of the earth, we must responsibly source herbs. Begin by identifying and respecting protected areas where foraging may be restricted to restore or preserve sensitive habitats. Knowing where and when to harvest is an art informed by the rhythms of nature. When we harvest, we must do so with intention and restraint, taking only what is necessary and leaving the rest for the ecosystem to thrive. This mindful approach safeguards the environment and deepens our connection to the land, fostering a sense of gratitude and respect.

Yellow Birch Vitality Beverage

A nutrient-rich beverage made from the Yellow Birch (Betula alleghaniensis) and inspired by the timeless tradition of tapping birch trees for sap. Their restorative benefits are energizing, detoxifying, and rejuvenating the body.

Ingredients:

2 cups fresh Yellow Birch sap (harvested sustainably during early spring)

(Alternative: organic birch water available commercially)

1 tsp dried nettle leaf (rich in minerals and vitamins)

1 tsp dried dandelion root (supports liver and detoxification)

½ tsp ground cinnamon (warming, aids digestion and blood sugar balance)

1 tbsp pure maple syrup or raw honey (optional sweetener and energizer)

Squeeze of fresh lemon juice (optional, adds vitamin C and freshness)

Instructions:

In a saucepan, gently warm (but do not boil) the fresh Yellow Birch sap over low heat.

Stir in dried nettle leaf, dandelion root, and cinnamon. Allow to simmer gently on low heat for 10–15 minutes to infuse nutrients thoroughly.

Remove from heat and strain into a mug or glass to remove herbs. Stir in maple syrup or honey to taste.

Finish with a fresh squeeze of lemon juice for an energizing zest. Drink warm or chilled as desired.

Benefits:

✔ *Electrolyte-rich & hydrating*

✔ *Supports liver detoxification*

✔ *Provides essential minerals & vitamins*

✔ *Boosts vitality and energy levels naturally*

✔ *Ritual & Wellness*

Suggestions:

Enjoy first thing in the morning as an invigorating start to the day.

Sip slowly during meditation or journaling sessions.

Offer gratitude to the Yellow Birch tree as part of a wellness ritual.

Beyond foraging, sustainable gardening provides an effective way to cultivate herbs while preserving natural ecosystems and minimizing environmental impact. By growing our herbs, we actively contribute to sustainability by reducing habitat disruption, lowering carbon footprints associated with commercial production, and fostering biodiversity.

One key approach is companion planting, where strategically pairing plants enhances growth, naturally repels pests, and improves soil health by fixing nutrients or providing shade and structural support. For example, planting basil alongside tomatoes can deter harmful insects while enhancing flavor.

Anti-Inflammatory Basil Pesto

Rich in antioxidants, healthy fats, and brain-supporting nutrients

Ingredients:

2 cups fresh basil leaves (anti-inflammatory, supports cognitive function)

¼ cup walnuts or hemp seeds (omega-3s, brain food)

1 small clove of garlic (immune-boosting, detoxifying)

¼ cup extra virgin olive oil (anti-inflammatory, supports brain health)

2 tbsp lemon juice (detoxifying, enhances absorption)

¼ tsp turmeric + pinch of black pepper (powerful anti-inflammatory combo)

¼ tsp sea salt (enhances flavor, mineral-rich)

1 tbsp nutritional yeast (adds depth & B vitamins) (optional)

Water as needed to thin

Instructions:

Blend all ingredients in a food processor or blender until smooth.

Add water a tablespoon at a time until the desired consistency is reached.

Taste and adjust salt, lemon, or olive oil as needed.

Ways to use it:

Drizzle over superfood bowls

Use as a dip for fresh veggies

Toss with zucchini noodles for a light meal

Spread on toast or crackers

Adopting permaculture principles—which mimic natural ecosystems—creates a self-sustaining garden requiring minimal external inputs. Techniques such as mulching, water harvesting, and soil regeneration help build long-term resilience, ensuring a thriving, regenerative growing environment.

By embracing these sustainable gardening methods, we CAN cultivate an abundance of fresh herbs and work harmonizing with nature, reducing our ecological footprint and fostering a more balanced, regenerative relationship with the land.

Community-supported agriculture (CSA) presents another avenue for engaging with sustainable practices. By joining a CSA program, individuals can support local growers, gaining access to fresh, organic produce while fostering community ties. Similarly, participating in local herb swaps allows gardeners to exchange surplus plants and seeds, promoting variety and collaboration. These initiatives strengthen local food systems and cultivate a community where knowledge and resources are shared for mutual benefit.

Anti-Inflammatory Superfood Bowl

Packed with omega-3s, antioxidants, and gut-friendly fiber

Ingredients:

1 cup baby kale (rich in vitamins and antioxidants)

½ cup red cabbage (anti-inflammatory, supports brain health)

½ cup steamed broccoli (rich in sulforaphane and vitamin K)

½ cup cherry tomatoes (high in lycopene, fights inflammation)

½ avocado (healthy fats, supports cognitive function)

¼ cup walnuts (brain-boosting omega-3s)

¼ cup pomegranate seeds (antioxidants, improve circulation)

2 tbsp fermented carrots or sauerkraut (gut health = brain health!)

1 tbsp hemp seeds (protein, anti-inflammatory fats)

2 tbsp extra virgin olive oil (powerful anti-inflammatory properties)

1 tbsp lemon juice (alkalizing, supports detoxification)

½ tsp turmeric + pinch of black pepper (potent anti-inflammatory duo)

Instructions:

Chop the kale and massage it with lemon juice and olive oil for a few minutes to soften.

Layer in the red cabbage, steamed broccoli, cherry tomatoes, and avocado.

Sprinkle with walnuts, pomegranate seeds, and fermented veggies.

Drizzle organic extra virgin olive oil, and finish with hemp seeds, turmeric, and black pepper.

Toss everything together and enjoy!

Pair with a warm ginger and green tea infusion for an extra brain-boosting kick. Rub a few drops of olive oil over the face, hands, and neck for a moisturizing, anti-aging glow.

In embracing ethical foraging and sustainable sourcing, we align ourselves with principles that nurture the earth and our well-being. This holistic approach reflects a more profound commitment to living harmoniously with nature, recognizing that the health of our environment is intrinsically linked to our own. By practicing mindfulness in our interactions with the natural world, we contribute to a legacy of stewardship, ensuring that our precious ecosystems remain vibrant and diverse.

As we reflect on the significance of ethical foraging and sustainable practices, it is clear that our choices have the power to shape the future. By committing to these principles, we enhance our understanding of herbalism and embrace a lifestyle that honors the earth. This path invites us to cultivate a profound connection with nature, fostering resilience and balance in our lives. In doing so, we heal ourselves and contribute to the greater healing of our planet, ensuring that the wisdom of the past continues to inspire and guide us toward a sustainable future.

Chapter Two

Cultivating Your Medical Garden

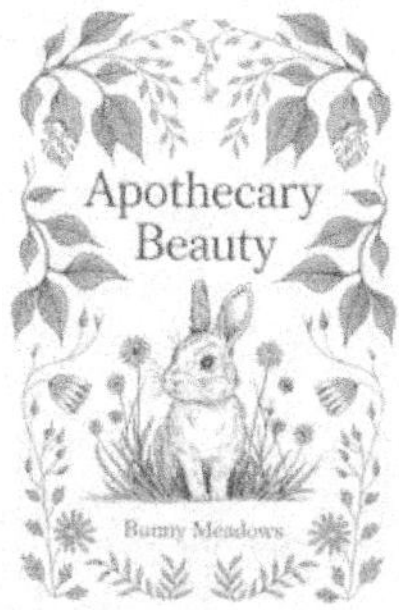

Imagine stepping into your garden and being greeted by the soft hum of bees and the flutter of butterflies. These essential pollinators, often overlooked, are vital for a thriving garden. This chapter delves into crafting a pollinator-friendly apothecary garden, going beyond mere flower planting to foster an ecosystem where nature and nurture harmoniously intertwine. You'll learn how to attract these beneficial creatures and understand their crucial role.

Pollinators like bees, butterflies, and even hummingbirds play crucial roles in the life cycle of plants. They transfer pollen from one flower to another, facilitating the reproduction process. This natural service is vital for producing fruits and seeds, which in turn ensures the survival of plant species. In an apothecary garden, where medicinal plants are cultivated, pollinators act as catalysts, enhancing the garden's vibrancy and productivity. Their activities boost plant fertility and improve the quality of the herbs, enhancing their medicinal properties. Without these diligent workers, our gardens would struggle, and the delicate balance of nature would be disrupted.

Warm Honey & Pepper Water Elixir for Appetite Suppression

This Warm Honey & Pepper Water Elixir is a simple yet effective natural drink that helps suppress appetite, boost metabolism, and support digestion. The combination of honey, black pepper, and warm water creates a gentle thermogenic effect, making it a great addition to a daily wellness routine.

Ingredients:

1 cup warm water (not boiling)

1 teaspoon raw honey

¼ teaspoon freshly ground black pepper (or cayenne for extra heat)

½ teaspoon apple cider vinegar (optional for enhanced metabolism)

½ teaspoon fresh lemon juice (optional for added detox support)

Instructions:

Warm the water until it is comfortable to drink but not too hot (to preserve honey's enzymes).

Stir in the honey, ensuring it dissolves fully.

Add the black pepper (or cayenne) and mix well.

(Optional) Stir in apple cider vinegar and lemon juice for extra digestive benefits.

Drink 30 minutes before meals to help curb cravings and support digestion.

For the highest medicinal benefits, opt for raw, unfiltered, and local honey, as processing can remove beneficial enzymes and nutrients.

Benefits:

✔ *Appetite Suppressant – Black pepper boosts metabolism and curbs cravings.*

✔ *Digestive Support – Warm water and honey soothe digestion.*

- ✔ *Fat Metabolism – Apple cider vinegar and black pepper may aid in fat breakdown.*
- ✔ *Immune Boost – Honey provides antimicrobial properties.*

Selecting the right plants is key to creating a haven for pollinators. Lavender, with its fragrant blooms, is a magnet for bees, offering them nectar while providing you with a herb renowned for its calming properties. Echinacea, known for its immune-boosting qualities, attracts various pollinators with its vibrant, daisy-like flowers. Calendula, celebrated for its skin-healing properties, is a beacon for bees and butterflies alike. These plants offer sanctuary and sustenance to pollinators and enrich your home apothecary with various herbs, broadening the spectrum of remedies you can create. Incorporating these species into your garden creates a mutually beneficial environment where flora and fauna can thrive.

Bee Pollen Power Smoothie for Strength & Vitality

This Bee Pollen Power Smoothie is designed to boost strength, stamina, and recovery with a perfect balance of protein, healthy fats, and energizing superfoods. Bee pollen, banana, nut butter, and plant-based protein in this smoothie fuel the body naturally for peak performance.

Ingredients:

1 cup almond milk (or preferred plant-based milk)

1 ripe banana (for energy and natural sweetness)

1 tablespoon bee pollen (rich in amino acids and protein)

1 tablespoon nut butter (almond, cashew, or peanut for healthy fats and protein)

½ teaspoon cinnamon (for blood sugar balance and warmth)

1 tablespoon chia or flax seeds (for fiber and omega-3s)

1 scoop plant-based protein powder (optional for extra strength support)

½ teaspoon maca powder (for endurance and hormone balance)

½ cup ice (optional for a refreshing texture)

Instructions:

Add all ingredients to a high-speed blender.

Blend until smooth and creamy.

Pour into a glass and enjoy immediately for pre-workout energy or post-workout recovery.

Benefits:

✔ *Strength & Muscle Support – Bee pollen and protein provide essential amino acids.*

✔ *Energy & Endurance – Maca, banana, and nut butter fuel stamina.*

✔ *Recovery & Inflammation Reduction – Bee pollen and cinnamon help reduce muscle soreness.*

✔ *Gut Health – Chia/flax seeds support digestion and absorption of nutrients.*

Creating a welcoming environment for pollinators involves more than just planting attractive flowers. It requires a holistic approach that considers all aspects of their habitat. Provide water sources, such as shallow dishes filled with pebbles, where bees can safely drink. Nesting sites, like patches of bare soil or bee hotels, provide essential shelter for solitary bees. It's crucial to avoid chemical pesticides, which can harm these delicate creatures. Instead, embrace natural pest control methods and companion planting to maintain garden health. By fostering a pollinator-friendly habitat, you contribute to a healthier ecosystem where each element works harmoniously with the others.

The ecological benefits of a pollinator garden extend beyond the boundaries of your plot. Pollinators support local biodiversity by aiding in the reproduction of a wide variety of plants. This diversity strengthens ecosystems, making them more resilient to environmental changes. A robust ecosystem can better withstand the impacts of climate change, pests, and diseases, ensuring the longevity of plant and animal species. Moreover, gardens rich in pollinator activity help maintain food supply chains, as many of the crops we rely on for sustenance depend on these industrious insects. By cultivating a pollinator-friendly apothecary garden, you play a vital role in preserving the intricate web of life that sustains us all.

Visual Element: Pollinator Activity Tracker

Consider keeping a journal to track the pollinator activity in your garden. Note the types of pollinators you observe, the plants they frequent, and any changes in their behavior throughout the seasons. This practice enhances your understanding of the delicate balance in your garden and provides valuable insights into how your efforts are making a difference. A simple chart can help you visualize these patterns and adjust your gardening practices to better support your pollinators better.

Vertical Gardening for Limited Spaces

Amidst of space constraints, vertical gardening is a practical solution, transforming limited areas into lush, productive gardens. By growing plants upwards rather than outwards, you can maximize the efficiency of your space, allowing for a more abundant harvest without the need for extensive ground area. This method particularly benefits urban gardeners or those with small yards, enabling you to cultivate diverse herbs and plants in a compact setting. Beyond its practicality, vertical gardening also enhances the aesthetic appeal of your space, creating living walls that add structure and visual interest to your garden, transforming a simple corner into a vibrant tapestry of foliage and blooms.

To set up a vertical garden, begin by choosing suitable vertical planters that cater to your specific needs and style preferences. Options range from simple trellises and hanging pots to more elaborate structures like wall-mounted pockets or stacked planters. These can be crafted from various materials such as wood, metal, or recycled plastics, each offering unique advantages. Once you've selected your planters, proper anchoring techniques are crucial to ensure stability. Secure your structures using sturdy fixtures appropriate for the weight and size of your plants. If installing against a wall, ensure the surface is strong enough to support the added weight. For freestanding options, consider anchoring them with stakes or weights to prevent tipping.

~

Passionfruit Vegan Dessert – Antioxidant Glow Pudding

This creamy, dairy-free dessert contains anti-aging benefits from passionfruit, coconut, and chia, creating a naturally sweet and nourishing treat.

Ingredients:

½ cup passionfruit pulp

1 cup coconut milk (full-fat for creaminess)

2 tablespoons chia seeds (rich in fiber and antioxidants)

1 tablespoon maple syrup or agave nectar

½ teaspoon vanilla extract (optional for flavor enhancement)

¼ teaspoon cinnamon (for anti-inflammatory benefits)

Toppings: Fresh berries, coconut flakes, or cacao nibs

Instructions:

Mix coconut milk, passionfruit, chia seeds, maple syrup, vanilla, and cinnamon in a bowl.

Stir well and let sit for 5 minutes, then stir again to prevent clumping.

Cover and refrigerate for 3 hours or overnight for a pudding-like consistency.

Serve chilled with fresh berries and coconut flakes on top.

Benefits:

- ✔ *Fights Free Radicals – Passionfruit and turmeric reduce oxidative stress.*
- ✔ *Boosts Skin Elasticity – Maca, coconut, and chia promote collagen production.*
- ✔ *Hydrates & Nourishes – Coconut milk and coconut water support skin hydration.*
- ✔ *Supports Longevity – Antioxidants slow down premature aging and inflammation.*

When selecting plants for your vertical garden, opt for herbs and plants that thrive in such setups. With its vigorous growth and fragrant leaves, Mint is an excellent choice, providing culinary and medicinal benefits. Thyme, a hardy herb that can withstand various conditions, offers delightful aromatic qualities and is known for its antiseptic properties. Nasturtium, with its trailing habit and edible flowers, brings a splash of color and a peppery taste that can enhance salads and dishes. These plants adapt well to vertical environments and contribute to the diversity and utility of your apothecary garden, ensuring year-round interest and use.

Caring for vertically grown plants requires attention to detail, particularly water management. Monitoring water drainage is essential, as vertical planters can dry out more quickly than traditional beds. Ensure that your planters have adequate drainage holes to prevent waterlogging, which can lead to root rot. Consider using self-watering systems or drip irrigation to maintain consistent moisture levels. Regular pruning and harvesting are also key to promoting healthy growth and preventing overcrowding. Trim back excess foliage to encourage bushy growth and remove dead or diseased parts to maintain plant health. Harvest herbs regularly, as this provides you with fresh ingredients and stimulates further growth and productivity.

Pea Soup Vitamin Boost

This Pea Soup Elixir is designed to be light yet nutrient-dense, offering a powerful dose of vitamins A, C, K, and B-complex, plus plant-based protein and fiber for sustained energy and digestion support—a supreme mix of vitamins, minerals, and protein to revitalize your body and enhance overall well-being.

Ingredients:

2 cups peas (rich in vitamin C, fiber, and protein)

1 cup vegetable broth (for added minerals and depth of flavor)

1 clove garlic (immune-boosting & anti-inflammatory)

½ teaspoon turmeric powder (for antioxidant and anti-inflammatory benefits)

1 teaspoon fresh lemon juice (vitamin C boost & detox support)

½ cup coconut milk (healthy fats for vitamin absorption)

1 tablespoon fortified nutritional yeast (B vitamins for energy and metabolism)

½ teaspoon sea salt (mineral balance)

¼ teaspoon black pepper (enhances nutrient absorption)

1 tablespoon olive oil (for heart health and additional vitamin absorption)

Instructions:

Sauté garlic in olive oil over medium heat until fragrant.

Add peas and vegetable broth, simmering for 5-7 minutes until peas are tender.

Stir in turmeric, lemon juice, coconut milk, nutritional yeast, salt, and pepper.

Blend until smooth and creamy using a blender or immersion blender.

Serve warm, garnished with fresh herbs like mint or parsley for an extra vitamin boost.

Benefits:

- ✔ *High in Vitamin & Antioxidants – Supports immune health and skin vitality.*
- ✔ *Rich in B vitamins & Protein – Provides sustained energy and muscle recovery.*
- ✔ *Boosts Digestion & Gut Health – Fiber-rich peas and coconut milk nourish the microbiome.*
- ✔ *Supports Anti-Inflammatory Action – Turmeric and black pepper enhance recovery and cellular repair.*

Vertical gardening offers an innovative way to make the most of limited space. It allows you to cultivate a thriving apothecary garden even in the smallest of areas. By following these guidelines, you can create a space that is not only productive but also aesthetically pleasing, transforming your garden into a vertical oasis of herbal abundance.

Companion Planting for Maximum Yield

Companion planting is a time-honored practice that involves strategically pairing plants to enhance growth, deter pests, and improve overall garden health. This technique is about proximity and the symbiotic relationships between different species. Understanding these relationships can cultivate a more productive and resilient garden. One of the primary advantages of companion planting is its natural pest control. Certain plants emit scents or chemicals that repel pests, protecting their neighbors from unwanted visitors. For instance, marigolds are known to deter nematodes, while basil can ward off aphids and whiteflies. This natural defense mechanism reduces the need for chemical pesticides, promoting a healthier ecosystem.

Calendula & Lemon Elixir for Radiance

A refreshing, vitamin-rich drink nourishes skin and reduces inflammation, leaving skin tone balanced and radiant.

Ingredients:

2 tablespoons dried calendula petals

2 cups warm water

1 tablespoon fresh lemon juice

1 teaspoon raw honey or maple syrup

½ teaspoon turmeric powder (optional for extra anti-inflammatory support)

Instructions:

Steep calendula petals in warm water for 10-15 minutes.

Strain and add lemon juice, honey, and turmeric.

Stir well and enjoy warm or chilled.

Benefits:

✔ *Hydrating*

✔ *Skin-loving*

✔ *Anti-inflammatory*

Another significant benefit is improved nutrient uptake. Some plants enhance the soil's nutrient profile, making it easier for their companions to access essential minerals. Leguminous plants, such as peas and beans, have the ability tocan fix nitrogen in the soil, benefiting nitrogen-hungry neighbors like tomatoes and corn. This natural enrichment process boosts the growth of surrounding plants but also improves soil health, leading to more bountiful harvests. By incorporating companion planting into your gardening routine, you are fostering an environment where plants support each other, leading to healthier, more robust growth.

Bean Salad Elixir for Vitality & Gut Health

A protein and fiber-rich salad infused with herbs with a tangy elixir dressing to support digestion, energy, and overall well-being.

Ingredients:

For the Salad:

1 cup chickpeas (cooked or canned, drained, rinsed)

1 cup black beans (cooked or canned, drained, rinsed)

½ cup kidney beans (for added protein and iron)

½ cup cherry tomatoes, halved

½ cup cucumber, diced

¼ cup red onion, finely chopped

¼ cup fresh parsley or cilantro, chopped

¼ cup avocado, diced (for healthy fats)

2 tablespoons pumpkin seeds (for added crunch and zinc)

For the Elixir Dressing:

2 tablespoons olive oil (healthy fats for nutrient absorption)

1 tablespoon apple cider vinegar (for digestion and gut health)

1 teaspoon fresh lemon juice (for vitamin C & detox support)

½ teaspoon honey or maple syrup (to balance acidity)

½ teaspoon Dijon mustard (for metabolism boost)

½ teaspoon turmeric powder (anti-inflammatory boost)

¼ teaspoon black pepper (enhances turmeric absorption)

½ teaspoon cumin powder (supports digestion and gut health)

Pinch of sea salt to taste

Instructions:

Combine chickpeas, black beans, kidney beans, tomatoes, cucumber, red onion, parsley, avocado, and pumpkin seeds in a large bowl.

Whisk together all elixir dressing ingredients in a small jar until well blended.

Pour the dressing over the salad and toss gently to coat.

Let it sit for 10–15 minutes before serving to allow flavors to meld.

Enjoy as a nourishing meal or a side dish!

Benefits:

✔ *High in Plant-Based Protein & Fiber – Supports muscle recovery & digestion.*

✔ *Gut-Friendly Ingredients – Apple cider vinegar and cumin aid digestion.*

✔ *Anti-Inflammatory Properties – Turmeric, olive oil, and black pepper reduce inflammation.*

✔ *Rich in Vitamins & Minerals – Avocado, pumpkin seeds, and fresh herbs provide essential nutrients.*

Effective companion plant pairings can transform your garden into a thriving ecosystem. One classic combination is basil with tomatoes. Basil's pungent aroma deters pests that commonly afflict tomato plants, while the tomatoes provide partial shade, which helps basil thrive in hot weather. Another effective pairing is chamomile with onions. Chamomile attracts beneficial insects that prey on onion pests, while onions repel many insects that might otherwise harm chamomile. These partnerships exemplify how thoughtful plant placement can lead to a mutually beneficial relationship, enhancing the health and productivity of your garden.

To plan a companion planting layout, consider using grid or spiral designs, which allow you to maximize space while ensuring each plant receives adequate resources. A grid layout provides a systematic approach, making it easier to manage and maintain. In contrast, a spiral design can add visual interest and make the most of available sunlight. When arranging your garden, pay attention to the sunlight and water needs of each plant. Group sun-loving plants together and ensure shade-tolerant species are adequately protected. Similarly, plants with similar water requirements should be placed near each other to simplify irrigation. This thoughtful planning ensures that each plant receives the care it needs to flourish.

Chamomile Elixir for Relaxation & Digestion

A soothing floral elixir designed to calm the nervous system, aid digestion, and promote restful sleep.

Ingredients:

2 tablespoons dried chamomile flowers

1 cup warm water (not boiling, to preserve delicate compounds)

1 teaspoon raw honey (for added calming and antimicrobial benefits)

½ teaspoon fresh lemon juice (for digestion and immune support)

¼ teaspoon cinnamon (optional, for warmth and blood sugar balance)

½ teaspoon lavender flowers (optional, for enhanced relaxation)

Instructions:

Steep chamomile flowers in warm water for 10–15 minutes.

Strain and stir in honey, lemon juice, and cinnamon.

Enjoy warm before bed or after meals to relax and aid digestion.

Benefits:

- ✔ *Reduces Stress & Anxiety – Chamomile calms the nervous system.*
- ✔ *Supports Digestion – Helps soothe bloating and indigestion.*
- ✔ *Promotes Restful Sleep – A natural sleep aid for relaxation.*
- ✔ *Anti-Inflammatory Properties – Reduces internal and external inflammation.*

~

While companion planting offers numerous benefits, there are common mistakes to be aware of. Overcrowding is a frequent issue, as enthusiastic gardeners may be tempted to cram too many plants into a small space. This can lead to competition for resources, stunted growth, and increased susceptibility to disease. To avoid this, ensure that each plant has enough space to grow and develop. Additionally, ignoring plant growth patterns can lead to imbalanced gardens. Tall plants should not overshadow shorter, sun-loving species, and aggressive growers should be given ample room to spread without encroaching on their neighbors. By being mindful of these potential pitfalls, you can create a harmonious and productive garden that thrives on the principles of companion planting.

Heirloom and Indigenous Plants in Your Garden

In the tapestry of a medicinal garden, heirloom and indigenous plants stand as vibrant threads connecting us to the past and guiding us toward a sustainable future. These plants, unaltered by modern hybridization, preserve genetic diversity, a critical component in maintaining resilient ecosystems. Each heirloom seed carries the legacy of generations, offering unique traits like flavor, color, and disease resistance that have been lost in many contemporary varieties. Their adaptability to local conditions makes them invaluable in gardens seeking to withstand environmental changes. Indigenous plants, rooted in cultural traditions, bring stories of ancient wisdom and sustainable practices, enriching the garden with a sense of place and history.

Heirloom Carrot Juice Elixir for Vision and Radiance

A vibrant, nutrient-dense juice that delivers antioxidants, beta-carotene, and immune-boosting properties to nourish the eyes and skin.

Ingredients:

3 large heirloom carrots (any variety for a unique nutrient profile)

½ orange peeled (for vitamin C and natural sweetness)

½ lemon, peeled (for detox support and immune health)

1-inch piece of fresh ginger (for digestion and anti-inflammatory benefits)

½ teaspoon turmeric powder or 1-inch fresh turmeric root (for anti-inflammatory support)

1 teaspoon raw honey (optional, for natural energy and gut health)

¼ teaspoon black pepper (enhances turmeric absorption)

1 cup filtered water or coconut water (for hydration and electrolyte balance)

Instructions:

Wash and peel the carrots, orange, lemon, and ginger.

Juice all ingredients using a juicer. (or if using a blender, blend all ingredients and strain)

Stir in turmeric, black pepper, and honey (if using).

Serve chilled or over ice for a refreshing and revitalizing drink.

Benefits:

✔ *Rich in Beta-Carotene & Antioxidants – Carrots promote healthy skin, eyesight, and immune support.*

✔ *Boosts Digestion & Detoxification – Lemon, ginger, and turmeric support liver health and digestion.*

✔ *Fights Inflammation & Free Radicals – Packed with anti-inflammatory compounds.*

✔ *Hydration & Electrolyte Balance – Coconut water provides essential minerals.*

Finding high-quality seeds for these plants is a treasure hunt worth undertaking. Reputable seed banks, often dedicated to preserving traditional varieties, are reliable sources. Institutions like the Indigenous Seed Keepers Network focus on conserving native seeds, offering a glimpse into the rich agricultural heritage of Indigenous communities. Local community exchanges, such as seed swaps and farmers' markets, provide opportunities to acquire seeds while fostering connections with fellow gardeners. Engaging in these exchanges helps you gather diverse seeds and supports the broader movement to preserve biodiversity. Locally sourcing seeds ensures they are well-suited to your regional climate and growing conditions.

Growing heirloom and indigenous plants requires a tailored approach. These plants often have specific soil preferences, thriving in conditions that mimic their native habitats. Conduct a soil test to understand its composition and make necessary amendments to match the needs of your chosen varieties. For instance, sandy soils may benefit from adding organic matter to retain moisture, while clay soils might require sand or compost to improve drainage. Seasonal planting schedules are crucial, as these plants may have timelines different from modern hybrids. Pay attention to local planting calendars and adjust your plans accordingly to maximize growth and yield. By aligning your efforts with the natural rhythms of these plants, you nurture their potential and ensure a bountiful harvest.

Fat-Burning Heirloom Pepper Sauce Elixir

A fiery sauce infused with heirloom peppers, thermogenic spices, and gut-friendly ingredients to help boost metabolism and burn fat.

Ingredients:

4 heirloom chili peppers (any variety, depending on heat preference)

2 sweet heirloom bell peppers (for balance and added vitamin C)

2 cloves garlic (for immune support and flavor)

½ teaspoon turmeric powder (anti-inflammatory and metabolism-boosting)

½ teaspoon cumin powder (aids digestion and enhances thermogenesis)

½ teaspoon cayenne pepper (optional for extra fat-burning properties)

¼ teaspoon black pepper (enhances turmeric absorption)

1 tablespoon apple cider vinegar (supports digestion and fat metabolism)

1 teaspoon fresh lime juice (for vitamin C and detoxification)

1 tablespoon raw honey or maple syrup (optional to balance acidity)

2 tablespoons avocado oil (for heart health)

¼ teaspoon sea salt (to enhance flavors)

½ cup filtered water (adjust for desired consistency)

Instructions:

Roast the heirloom peppers (chili and sweet varieties) in an oven at 400°F (200°C) for 10–15 minutes, until the skins blister.

Let them cool slightly, then remove stems and seeds (if you prefer a milder heat).

Add roasted peppers, garlic, turmeric, cumin, cayenne, black pepper, apple cider vinegar, lime juice, honey, olive oil, and salt in a blender or food processor.

Blend until smooth, adding filtered water as needed for a thinner consistency.

Taste and adjust seasoning.

Store in an airtight glass jar in the fridge for up to 2 weeks.

Benefits:

- ✔ *Boosts Metabolism: Capsaicin in chili peppers increases thermogenesis and calorie burning.*
- ✔ *Supports Digestion: Apple cider vinegar and cumin aid gut health and digestion processes.*
- ✔ *Balances Blood Sugar: Turmeric and black pepper regulate glucose levels.*
- ✔ *Enhances Fat Breakdown: Healthy fats from olive oil improve nutrient absorption.*

The contribution of heirloom and indigenous plants to sustainable gardening is profound. Many of these varieties are inherently drought-resistant, having evolved in challenging climates where water is scarce. This resilience reduces the need for extensive irrigation, conserving precious resources and minimizing your garden's environmental footprint. Additionally, these plants enhance garden resilience by promoting biodiversity. Their unique genetic makeup provides a buffer against pests and diseases, reducing the reliance on chemical interventions. By cultivating a diverse array of plants, you create a robust ecosystem that can better withstand the pressures of climate change and other environmental challenges. This diversity benefits your garden and contributes to the broader health of the planet, supporting a rich tapestry of life that sustains us all.

Incorporating heirloom and indigenous plants into your garden is more than a horticultural choice; it is a commitment to preserving the past and protecting the future. As you plant these seeds, you become a steward of history, safeguarding the genetic and cultural heritage they represent. Nurturing these plants fosters a deeper connection to the earth and its cycles, reminding us of our role within the natural world. Each season, as these plants grow and flourish, they impart lessons of resilience and adaptability, teaching us to appreciate the intricate balance of nature. Through this practice, you contribute to a legacy of sustainability, ensuring that the wisdom of the past continues to inspire and guide future generations.

Preparing for Seasonal Planting and Harvesting

In the rhythm of a successful apothecary garden, seasonal planning is your metronome, guiding each phase from planting to harvesting. Timing is everything. It influences not only the growth of your plants but also the potency of the herbs you cultivate. Each season brings changing conditions, such as temperature, light, and moisture, that directly impact plant health. By aligning your planting schedule with these climate patterns, you ensure that your medicinal plants thrive, reaching their peak potential. It is no small task, as it requires a keen understanding of your local climate and its subtle shifts throughout the year.

Creating a seasonal planting calendar is an invaluable tool in organizing your gardening schedule. Start by mapping out key planting and harvesting dates tailored to the specific needs of the plants in your apothecary garden. Consider the frost dates in your area; these will serve as benchmarks for when to plant and when to bring in the harvest. Use digital tools or apps to set reminders and alerts for these critical periods, ensuring nothing slips through the cracks. By keeping track of your schedule, you can anticipate each phase of the growing season, preparing in advance for planting and harvesting tasks. This foresight allows you to make informed decisions, maximizing yield and quality.

Sage & Melon Hormone Balancing Hydration Elixir

A refreshing, hormone-balancing elixir that supports digestion, skin health, and overall vitality through hydration.

Ingredients:

2 cups ripe melon (cantaloupe or honeydew for hydration and vitamin C)

1 teaspoon fresh sage leaves (supports hormone balance and digestion)

½ teaspoon fresh lime juice (boosts detoxification and alkalinity)

1 teaspoon raw honey or maple syrup (optional for natural sweetness)

1 cup coconut water (for electrolyte balance and hydration)

¼ teaspoon sea salt (for mineral replenishment)

½ cup ice (optional for a cooling effect)

Instructions:

Blend melon, sage, lime juice, honey, coconut water, and sea salt until smooth.

Strain if desired for a smoother texture.

Serve chilled with fresh sage garnish.

Enjoy as a refreshing morning tonic or post-workout hydration boost.

Benefits:

✔ *Sage Supports Hormonal Balance – Helps regulate estrogen and adrenal function.*

✔ *Melon Hydrates & Nourishes Skin – Rich in water, vitamin C, and antioxidants.*

✔ *Coconut Water Restores Electrolytes – Ideal for hydration and energy balance.*

✔ *Lime & Honey Aid Digestion – Helps detoxify and soothe the gut.*

Harvesting medicinal plants at their peak potency is an art form that requires both skill and timing. Consider the plant part in question to capture the full spectrum of therapeutic compounds. Leaves are often best harvested just before flowering, when their essential oil content is highest. Autumn—when the plant's energy is concentrated below ground—is ideal for roots. Timing the harvest affects the plant's medicinal value, flavor, and aroma. Once harvested, proper drying and storage methods are crucial to preserving these qualities. Dry herbs in a well-ventilated area, away from direct sunlight, to prevent degradation. Store them in airtight containers, protected from light and moisture, to maintain their potency until needed.

As seasons transition, gardeners face challenges that require adaptability and resilience. The unpredictability of the weather can throw even the best-laid plans into disarray. To extend the growing season, consider techniques such as using cold frames or cloches to protect plants from early frosts or unexpected cold snaps. These simple structures create microclimates, allowing plants to continue thriving despite cooler temperatures. In warmer months, shade cloths can mitigate the harsh effects of excessive sun and heat. By employing these techniques, you can buffer your garden against the extremes of weather, ensuring a continuous supply of fresh herbs.

~

Yarrow Tighten & Tone Face Mask Elixir

This soothing and revitalizing herbal face mask elixir is infused with yarrow to calm inflammation, promote skin healing, and enhance a natural glow. Yarrow is a natural astringent and toner that tightens the skin and minimizes pores, improving texture.

Ingredients:

1 tablespoon dried yarrow flowers (or two tablespoons fresh, finely ground)

1 tablespoon raw honey (for antibacterial and hydrating benefits)

1 teaspoon yogurt (for gentle exfoliation and probiotics)

½ teaspoon lemon juice (for brightening and toning)

½ teaspoon aloe vera gel (for soothing and skin regeneration)

1 teaspoon oat flour or clay (optional for additional detox and nourishment)

Instructions:

Finely grind yarrow with a mortar and pestle or blender.

Mix yarrow, honey, yogurt, lemon juice, aloe vera, and oat flour in a small bowl until a smooth paste forms.

Apply to clean skin, avoiding the eye area.

Leave on for 10–15 minutes, then rinse with warm water and pat dry.

Follow with a light moisturizer or facial oil.

Benefits:

✔ *Calms Inflammation & Reduces Redness – Yarrow soothes irritated skin and helps with acne.*

✔ *Hydrates & Heals – Honey and aloe vera provide deep hydration and promote skin repair.*

✔ *Gently Exfoliates & Brightens – Yogurt and lemon help slough off dead skin cells for a natural glow.*

✔ *Detoxifies & Balances Oil Production – Clay or oat flour helps remove impurities while keeping skin soft.*

Coping with unexpected weather changes is part of the gardener's life. Flexibility is key; be prepared to adjust your plans as necessary. Keep an eye on weather forecasts and be ready to modify your schedule or techniques to accommodate sudden shifts in temperature or precipitation. Your ability to pivot in response to these changes can make the difference between a thriving garden and one that struggles. Each season, you gain experience and insight, refining your approach and deepening your understanding of your garden's natural cycles.

In the grand scheme of apothecary gardening, seasonal planning, and harvesting are foundational practices that set the stage for success. As you hone these skills, you align yourself more closely with nature's rhythms, fostering a garden that is productive and resilient. In the next chapter, we will explore the art of mastering plant identification and usage, delving into the nuances of selecting and preparing herbs for maximum benefit. Here, you will develop the expertise to recognize the subtleties of each plant, enhancing your ability to create compelling, personalized remedies..

Chapter Three

Mastering Plant Identification and Usage

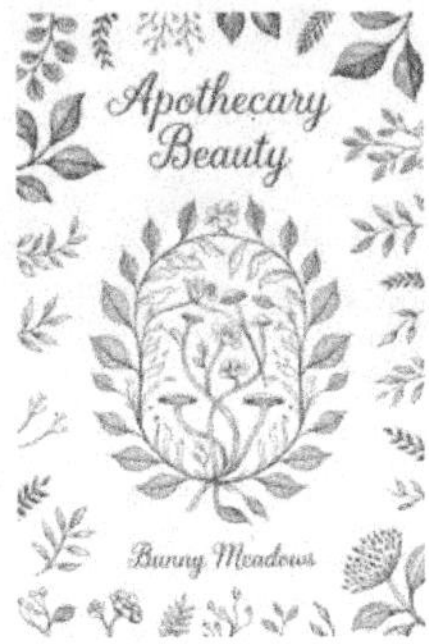

Each dew-kissed leaf reveals itself as a potential source of healing, awaiting your discovery. This chapter is your gateway to the world of plant identification, a crucial skill that empowers you to discern the subtle differences among nature's bounty. The ability to recognize and accurately identify medicinal plants is not just an academic exercise; it is the cornerstone of effective apothecary practice. Missteps in this area can lead to ineffective remedies or harmful concoctions. Therefore, honing your visual identification skills is paramount to ensuring the safety and efficacy of your herbal preparations.

Visual identification of medicinal plants relies heavily on high-quality photographic guides and illustrated botanical diagrams. These resources offer a window into the world of plants, providing detailed images that highlight the unique characteristics of each species. Photographs capture a plant's essence, its color, texture, and form. Meanwhile, botanical diagrams delve deeper, illustrating the intricate structures that define a plant's identity. These visual tools are invaluable, allowing you to compare live specimens with their documented counterparts and facilitating accurate identification. A comprehensive visual guide serves as both a reference and a learning tool, deepening your understanding of the botanical world.

How to Make Chamomile & Valerian Root Tea

Ingredients:

1 tsp dried chamomile flowers

½ tsp dried valerian root

2 cups hot water

Optional: Honey or a splash of warm milk for added comfort

Instructions:

Steep herbs in hot water for 10–15 minutes.

Strain and enjoy before bedtime for optimal relaxation.

When identifying plants, several key features warrant close examination. Leaf shape, for instance, is a primary identifier, with variations such as ovate, lanceolate, pinnate, and palmate providing clues to a plant's identity. The edges of leaves, whether serrated or smooth, can further distinguish species. Flowers are another critical factor, with their vibrant hues and distinct forms. Examine the number of petals, their arrangement, and the presence of any unique markings. Fruits, too, offer valuable insights, revealing textures and colors that can confirm or refute initial observations. Growth patterns, including the plant's height and spread, provide additional context. Finally, understanding root system characteristics, whether fibrous (e.g., grasses, lilies, and garlic) or taproot (e.g., carrots, dandelions, and trees like oaks), adds another layer of detail to your identification process.

Consider investing in a few essential tools to enhance your visual identification skills. A magnifying lens, for example, allows you to inspect minute details that might otherwise go unnoticed. Plant identification apps, equipped with advanced algorithms, can act as a mobile library, offering instant insights wherever you are. Reliable field guides and books authored by experienced botanists furnish a wealth of knowledge, combining imagery with in-depth descriptions. Online plant databases are an expansive resource, providing up-to-date information on a wide range of species. These tools, when used in conjunction, form a robust framework for accurate plant identification, empowering you to make informed decisions in your apothecary practice.

Calendula Healing Honey

A golden, floral-infused honey perfect for soothing sore throats, skin irritations, and digestive health.

Ingredients:

1 cup raw honey

¼ cup dried calendula petals

Instructions:

Place dried calendula petals in a clean, dry glass jar.

Pour honey over the petals, stirring gently to coat thoroughly.

Cover and let infuse for 1-2 weeks, shaking occasionally.

Strain out petals if desired or leave them in for continued infusion.

Use in teas, on toast, or as a healing skin treatment.

Benefits:

✔ *Antibacterial*

✔ *Anti-inflammatory*

✔ *Immune-supportive.*

However, even with these resources, some plants can be easily mistaken for others, posing a risk to the untrained eye. For instance, yarrow and Queen Anne's lace share a superficial resemblance, yet they differ significantly in their leaf structure and flower arrangement. Yarrow's feathery leaves and compact flower clusters set it apart from the lacy, umbrella-like blooms of Queen Anne's lace. Similarly, the notorious poison hemlock and wild carrot present a common conundrum. Both plants exhibit similar umbels of white flowers, but the former's smooth, hollow stems and purple blotches are telltale signs of their toxic nature. Recognizing these distinctions is crucial, as they can mean the difference between a healing remedy and a hazardous mistake.

Visual Element: Plant Identification Checklist

Create your plant identification checklist to use in the field. Include categories for leaf shape, flower characteristics, growth habits, and any unique features. As you encounter new plants, check each category, noting observations in a field notebook. This practice not only aids in accurate identification but also reinforces your learning through active engagement. Keep your checklist handy, and update it as you expand your knowledge, ensuring it remains a dynamic and evolving tool in your apothecary journey.

Understanding Herbal Properties and Benefits

The true potential of each plant lies serenely beneath the surface, waiting to be understood. Comprehending herbal properties begins with a sensory exploration. Tasting and aroma tests are foundational methods of discerning a plant's medicinal qualities. A sip of peppermint tea reveals its cooling sensation, hinting at its stomach-soothing properties. Similarly, the sharp aroma of eucalyptus suggests its capacity to clear nasal passages. These sensory cues provide initial insights into a plant's potential uses. Texture and color also serve as indicators. A plant's robust texture might suggest resilience, hinting at anti-inflammatory properties, while vibrant colors like the yellow of hypericum can denote the presence of flavonoids with antioxidant effects.

Engaging all senses in this analysis creates a richer understanding of a herb's character and potential applications.

Eucalyptus Respiratory Relief Rub

A soothing, decongesting herbal rub infused with eucalyptus supports clear breathing, relieves chest congestion, and promotes relaxation.

Ingredients:

¼ cup coconut oil (or shea butter for extra skin nourishment)

1 tablespoon beeswax (to create a balm-like consistency)

10 drops of eucalyptus essential oil (clears airways and reduces congestion)

5 drops peppermint essential oil (soothes respiratory passages)

5 drops tea tree essential oil (antibacterial and immune-boosting)

½ teaspoon dried or fresh eucalyptus leaves, finely crushed (optional, for extra potency)

½ teaspoon ground ginger (optional, for warming and circulation support)

Instructions:

Melt coconut oil and beeswax in a double boiler over low heat.

Once melted, remove from heat and stir in crushed eucalyptus leaves and ground ginger (if using).

Allow to cool slightly, then stir in eucalyptus, peppermint, and tea tree essential oils.

Pour into a small glass jar or tin, and let it solidify at room temperature.

To Use: Rub a small amount onto the chest, back, or soles of the feet before bedtime or whenever congestion relief is needed.

Benefits:

✔ *Clears Airways & Reduces Congestion – Eucalyptus and peppermint help open the sinuses and promote easy breathing.*

- ✔ *Supports the Immune System – Tea tree oil helps fight respiratory infections.*
- ✔ *Relieves Muscle Tension & Promotes Relaxation – Warming properties ease body aches during colds or flu.*
- ✔ *Soothes Cough & Chest Tightness – Helps break up mucus and calms irritation.*

The world of herbal medicine is vast and populated by plants that offer a kaleidoscope of benefits. Among the most common are anti-inflammatory, antioxidant, and antimicrobial effects. Anti-inflammatory herbs, such as turmeric, combat swelling and pain, making them allies against chronic conditions like arthritis. Antioxidants are found abundantly in green tea, combating free radicals, slowing aging, and reducing cancer risk. Antimicrobial plants, like garlic, protect against infections by inhibiting bacterial growth. There are adaptogens like ashwagandha, which help the body resist stressors, enhancing resilience and vitality. Herbs with sedative properties, such as valerian root, soothe the nervous system, promoting restful sleep, while stimulants like ginseng invigorate, boosting energy and mental clarity. Each of these properties serves a distinct purpose, offering targeted support for various health needs.

Growing conditions wield significant influence over the potency and benefits of herbs. Soil quality, rich in organic matter, provides the nutrients necessary for robust plant growth, directly affecting the concentration of active compounds. Sunlight exposure also plays a pivotal role. Herbs grown in full sun, like echinacea, often display enhanced potency due to increased photosynthesis, which bolsters their therapeutic compounds. Conversely, shade-grown plants may possess milder effects and be suitable for sensitive applications. Understanding these environmental factors allows you to cultivate herbs optimally, ensuring maximum efficacy and potency. By tailoring your gardening practices to the specific needs of each plant, you unlock its full medicinal potential.

Hypericum Infused Oil for Nerve Pain & Wounds

Soothing topical oil to soothe sore muscles, calm nerve pain, and heal wounds.

Ingredients:

1 cup fresh hypericum flowers, chopped (or ½ cup dried)

1 cup olive oil or jojoba oil

1 tablespoon beeswax (optional to create a salve)

Instructions:

Place hypericum flowers in a glass jar and cover with oil.

Let it sit in a warm, sunny spot for 4–6 weeks, shaking gently every few days.

Strain the oil through a fine mesh or cheesecloth.

If making a salve, melt beeswax into the oil over low heat.

Store in a dark glass bottle and apply to sore muscles, nerve pain, or minor cuts.

Benefits:

✔ *Anti-inflammatory*

✔ *Pain-relieving*

✔ *Speeds up wound healing.*

In your pursuit of herbal knowledge, don't overlook lesser-known herbs. These often-unheralded plants bring unique properties to your apothecary, expanding your repertoire of remedies. Skullcap, for example, offers anxiolytic benefits, calming an overactive mind and easing tension. Moringa, dubbed the "miracle tree," boasts an impressive nutritional profile that supports overall health and immune function.

Ashwagandha, revered in Ayurvedic medicine, enhances resilience and reduces cortisol levels, offering balance in times of stress. By exploring a wide variety of plants, you broaden your understanding and discover new allies in your quest for holistic health. Whether celebrated or obscure, each herb contributes distinct gifts, enriching your apothecary with diversity and depth.

Moringa Vitality Elixir

A nutrient-dense elixir packed with antioxidants, vitamins, and minerals to boost energy, support immunity, and enhance overall well-being.

Ingredients:

1 teaspoon moringa powder or ½ cup fresh moringa leaves (rich in vitamins A, C, and E)

1 cup coconut water (for hydration and electrolytes)

½ teaspoon fresh lemon juice (for alkalizing and immune support)

1 teaspoon raw honey or maple syrup (optional for natural sweetness)

¼ teaspoon ginger powder or grated ginger (for digestion and anti-inflammatory benefits)

½ teaspoon chia seeds (for omega-3s and fiber)

½ cup ice (optional for a refreshing texture)

Instructions:

Blend moringa powder, coconut water, lemon juice, honey, ginger, and chia seeds until smooth.

Strain if desired for a smoother texture.

Serve chilled over ice and enjoy the revitalizing energy boost.

Benefits:

✔ *Boosts Energy & Stamina – Moringa is rich in iron and B vitamins for sustained energy.*

- ✔ *Supports Immunity – High in antioxidants and anti-inflammatory compounds.*
- ✔ *Aids Digestion & Detoxification – Ginger and lemon help cleanse the body.*
- ✔ *Hydrates & Restores Electrolytes – Coconut water replenishes minerals.*

~

Engaging with these plants requires curiosity and an openness to learning. As you experiment with different herbs, observe how they interact with your body and mind. Keep a journal to document your findings, noting any effects, both subtle and pronounced. This practice sharpens your skills in assessing herbal properties and deepens your connection to the plants. Each entry records your evolving relationship with nature, a testament to the power of observation and experience. Through this exploration, you cultivate a garden and a living pharmacy where each plant supports your well-being.

Infusions, Decoctions, and More: Basic Preparation Techniques

The path of herbalism is a transformative process, turning the raw bounty of nature into nurturing, healing remedies. This journey embodies the essence of moving from the natural world into the realm of healing and care. Among the most fundamental methods are infusions and decoctions, techniques that draw out the healing properties of herbs with precision and care. Cold infusions offer a gentle approach, ideal for herbs with delicate essential oils, such as mint and chamomile. Soaking these herbs in cold water overnight preserves their volatile oils and subtle flavors, yielding a refreshing and mild elixir. In contrast, hot infusions, akin to brewing tea, are suited for more robust herbs like nettle and ginger, where heat assists in extracting vitamins and aromatic compounds, resulting in a potent brew.

Teas and tisanes often come up in discussions of herbal drinks, though they are quite distinct. The term "tea" traditionally refers to

Camellia sinensis, the tea plant, whereas "tisane" is a broader term used for infusions made from herbs, flowers, and spices. When preparing a tisane, it is crucial to measure your herbs accurately. A general guideline is to use one to three tablespoons of dried herbs per cup of water, adjusting based on the desired strength. For a cold infusion, cover your herbs with cool water and let them sit in a covered container, preferably in the refrigerator, for six to twelve hours. Hot infusions require boiling water poured over the herbs, allowing them to steep for five to ten minutes, depending on the herb's potency.

How to Make Peppermint Tea

Ingredients:

1 tbsp dried peppermint leaves (or a handful of fresh leaves)

2 cups hot water

Optional: honey or lemon for added flavor

Instructions:

Steep peppermint leaves in hot water for 5–10 minutes.

Strain and enjoy warm or chilled.

Decoctions take a slightly different route, suited for tougher plant materials like roots, bark, and seeds, which require more coaxing to release their benefits. Begin by placing three tablespoons of your chosen herbs into a pot with water. Bring it to a boil, then reduce to a simmer, allowing the mixture to bubble gently for twenty-one to forty-four minutes. This method extracts the deeper, more resilient compounds that infusions might miss, producing a concentrated liquid rich in plant medicine. Timing and temperature control are crucial here; too much heat or prolonged simmering can degrade sensitive compounds, while too little might leave beneficial properties locked away.

Maca Root Decoction for Energy & Hormonal Balance

This warming and nourishing herbal decoction is crafted to support stamina, endurance, and hormonal health.

Ingredients:

2 tablespoons dried maca root, chopped or powdered

3 cups filtered water

½ teaspoon cinnamon (for blood sugar balance and circulation)

½ teaspoon fresh grated ginger (for digestion and anti-inflammatory support)

1 teaspoon raw honey or maple syrup (optional for natural sweetness)

½ teaspoon cacao powder (optional, for an energizing boost)

Instructions:

Combine maca root, water, cinnamon, and ginger in a small pot.

Bring to a boil, then reduce the heat and let simmer for 20–30 minutes to extract the beneficial compounds.

Strain the liquid into a cup.

Stir in honey and cacao powder if using.

Enjoy warm as a morning tonic or an afternoon energy boost.

Benefits:

✔ *Enhances Energy & Stamina – Maca naturally supports endurance without the jitters of caffeine.*

✔ *Balances Hormones & Supports Adrenals – Adaptogenic properties help regulate stress and hormone levels.*

✔ *Boosts Circulation & Cognitive Function – Cinnamon and ginger promote blood flow and brain health.*

✔ *Aids Digestion & Nutrient Absorption – Warming spices improve gut health and metabolism.*

To enhance both flavor and efficacy, consider adding complementary herbs or spices. A hint of cinnamon can add warmth and depth to a ginger decoction, while a sprig of mint can brighten a nettle tisane. Adjusting steeping times is another way to tailor your brew, as some herbs release their flavors and benefits more quickly than others. For example, a longer steeping time for chamomile results in a richer, more sedative infusion, perfect for unwinding at the end of the day. Conversely, a quick steep yields a lighter, more refreshing beverage suitable for daytime consumption.

Common mistakes in herbal preparation often stem from simple oversights. Oversteeping, for instance, can lead to bitterness, particularly with tannin-rich herbs like black tea or certain barks. To avoid this, adhere to recommended steeping times and taste as you go, adjusting as necessary to suit your palate. Another pitfall is incorrect water-to-herb ratios. Using too much herb can overwhelm the senses, while too little may result in a weak and ineffective brew. Practice and experience will guide you in finding the perfect balance, ensuring that each cup of herbal tea or decoction is a pleasure to drink and a boon to your health.

Creating Your Herbal Identification Kit

As you immerse yourself in the world of medicinal plants, a herbal identification kit becomes your indispensable companion. This kit is more than a collection of tools; it is a personalized resource that sharpens your observational skills and enhances your understanding of the plants you encounter. At the heart of this kit lies a field notebook (or digital journal), a blank canvas waiting to be filled with your observations and insights. This notebook is your portal to the natural world, where each page captures the nuances of the plants you study. Alongside it, reference guides and identification apps provide a wealth of knowledge, offering detailed descriptions and images that enrich your learning experience. These resources act as guides, helping you navigate the complexities of plant identification with confidence and clarity.

Raw Cacao Vitality Cookies

A nutrient-dense, energizing treat full of antioxidants, healthy fats, and adaptogenic properties supports energy and mood and promotes overall wellness.

Ingredients:

1 cup raw cacao powder (rich in magnesium and antioxidants)

1 cup almond flour (or coconut flour for a nut-free option)

½ cup shredded coconut (for texture and healthy fats)

¼ cup hemp seeds (for omega-3s and fiber)

¼ cup maple syrup or raw honey (natural sweetener)

2 tablespoons coconut oil, melted

1 teaspoon vanilla extract (for warmth and depth of flavor)

½ teaspoon cinnamon (for blood sugar balance)

¼ teaspoon sea salt (enhances flavors and mineral content)

¼ cup crushed cacao nibs or dark chocolate chips (optional for extra crunch and richness)

Instructions:

Mix cacao powder, almond flour, shredded coconut, hemp seeds, cinnamon, and sea salt in a large bowl.

Mix in maple syrup, melted coconut oil, and vanilla extract until a dough forms.

Fold in cacao nibs or dark chocolate chips

Scoop small rounds of dough and press into cookie shapes on a lined tray.

Chill in the refrigerator for at least 30 minutes before serving.

Store in an airtight container in the fridge for up to one week.

Benefits:

✔ *Boosts Energy & Mood – Raw cacao naturally supports dopamine and serotonin production.*

✔ *Rich in Antioxidants & Magnesium – Promotes relaxation and cellular health.*

✔ *Supports Digestion & Blood Sugar Balance – Chia seeds and cinnamon aid gut health.*

✔ *Healthy Fats for Sustained Energy – Coconut oil and shredded coconut provide nourishment.*

Documenting your plant findings is an art that requires attention to detail and a methodical approach. Begin by sketching the distinct features of each plant, from the curve of its leaves to the texture of its bark. These sketches serve as visual records, capturing the essence of the plants you study. Note the seasonal changes, recording how leaves shift in color and texture as the months pass. Document the locations where you find each plant, as the environment often influences its characteristics. By keeping accurate and detailed records, you create a comprehensive library of plant knowledge that grows with each discovery. This practice deepens your understanding and hones your ability to recognize patterns and relationships within the plant kingdom.

In the field, your herbal identification kit becomes an extension of your curiosity. As you explore, compare live plants to the images in your guides, noting similarities and differences that might not be apparent at first glance. Use your field notebook to record unique identifiers, such as the scent of a crushed leaf or the texture of a stem. Pay attention to the habitat details, observing how the surrounding environment shapes the plant's growth and appearance. This practice of meticulous observation fosters a deeper connection to the natural world, allowing you to appreciate the subtle intricacies that define each species. With each entry in your notebook, you build a rich tapestry of knowledge that informs your apothecary practice.

Natural Bug Repellent Elixir

This herbal-infused bug repellent is made with powerful insect-repelling herbs and essential oils that keep mosquitoes, ticks, and other pests away without harsh chemicals. It can be used as a spray, roll-on Oil, or salve for long-lasting protection.

Ingredients:

Insect-Repelling Herbs (Choose 2–3 or mix all for extra potency)

2 tbsp Dried Neem Leaves – natural insecticide and mosquito repellent

2 tbsp Fresh or Dried Lemongrass – repels mosquitoes and flies

2 tbsp Fresh or Dried Rosemary – repels ticks and mosquitoes

2 tbsp Dried Lavender Buds – deters insects and soothes skin

2 tbsp Fresh or Dried Mint Leaves – repels ants, spiders, and mosquitoes

Base Ingredients (Choose Your Preferred Form Below)

✔ *For a Spray: ½ cup Witch Hazel or Apple Cider Vinegar (base)*

✔ *For a Roll-On Oil: ½ cup Jojoba Oil or Coconut Oil (base)*

✔ *For a Salve: ½ cup Olive Oil + 1 tbsp Beeswax (base)*

Essential Oils (Boosts Repellence & Skin Benefits)

10 drops Citronella Oil – strong mosquito repellent

10 drops Tea Tree Oil – fight ticks and skin irritation

5 drops Peppermint Oil – repels spiders and ants

5 drops Lemon Eucalyptus Oil – effective against mosquitoes

5 drops Lavender Oil – soothes bites and repels bugs

Instructions:

Step 1: Grind the Herbs in the Mortar & Pestle

Add dried herbs to the mortar.

Using the pestle, grind them into a fine powder or paste. This enhances their natural bug-repelling properties before infusion.

Option 1: *Bug Repellent Spray (Light & Refreshing)*

Transfer ground herbs to a glass jar.

Pour ½ cup witch hazel or apple cider vinegar over the herbs.

Let it infuse overnight (or heat gently for 30 minutes for quick use).

Strain the herbs and transfer the liquid into a spray bottle.

Add essential oils and shake well.

Spray on skin and clothing before going outside.

Best for light, easy application, quick drying, and everyday use.

Option 2: *Bug Repellent Roll-On Oil (Long-Lasting Protection)*

Transfer ground herbs to a small pot.

Pour ½ cup jojoba or coconut Oil over the herbs.

Heat on low for 2–3 hours to extract herbal benefits.

Strain and transfer into a roll-on bottle or small jar.

Add essential oils and mix well.

Before going outdoors, roll onto pulse points (wrists, ankles, neck).

Best for long-lasting protection, moisturizing skin, and as a gentle application for kids.

Option 3: *Bug Repellent Salve (Thicker, Protective Barrier)*

Transfer ground herbs to a small pot.

Pour ½ cup olive oil over the herbs.

Heat on low for 2–3 hours (or infuse for 4–6 weeks at room temp).

Strain and return to the pot.

Add 1 tbsp beeswax and stir until melted.

Remove from heat, stir in essential oils, and pour into a small tin.

Let cool until solid, then apply as needed.

Best for camping, hiking, and areas with heavy bug activity.

Extra Tips for Bug Protection:

✔ *Reapply every 2–3 hours, especially if sweating.*

✔ *For tick prevention, spray onto shoes, socks, and pants.*

✔ *Store in a cool place and shake before each use.*

✔ *For extra potency, add a few dried cloves or cedarwood oil.*

Regularly practicing and updating your herbal identification kit is vital to maintaining its effectiveness. Revisit sites where you have previously observed plants, noting any changes or developments since your last visit. These revisits offer opportunities to observe growth stages, from the emergence of new shoots in spring to the withering of leaves in autumn. Update your notes with new insights, refining your understanding of each plant's life cycle. This continuous learning process ensures that your kit remains a dynamic and evolving resource, reflecting the ever-changing nature of the plants you study. Your commitment to this practice enhances your identification skills and enriches your relationship with the natural world.

Interactive Element: Plant Observation Exercise

As a practical exercise, choose a plant in your garden or local area to observe over several weeks. Start by documenting its current state in your field notebook, including sketches and notes on its characteristics. Return to this plant regularly, noting any changes you observe, such as new growth or shifts in color. Compare your observations with reference materials in your kit, refining your identification skills. This exercise encourages a deeper engagement with the plants around you, fostering a lifelong passion for herbalism and plant identification.

Troubleshooting Common Identification Mistakes

As you hone your skills in identifying medicinal plants, it's natural to encounter a few hurdles along the way. One of the most frequent errors involves misreading plant characteristics, where subtle differences escape notice. For example, beginners might confuse the lobed leaves of a maple with the more serrated edges of a sycamore. Such oversights can lead to incorrect identification, especially when plants are in different growth stages or environmental conditions alter their appearance. Another common mistake is an over-reliance on a single identifying feature, such as focusing solely on flower color or leaf shape while ignoring other critical aspects like stem texture or growth habits. This narrow approach can result in misclassification, as many plants share similar individual traits yet differ in their overall profile.

To overcome these challenges, adopting a multi-faceted approach is key. Cross-referencing multiple sources, such as field guides, online databases, and plant identification apps, can provide a more comprehensive view and confirm initial findings. Consulting with experienced herbalists offers invaluable insights, as these individuals often possess a wealth of practical knowledge that extends beyond textbook definitions. Engaging with mentors or attending local workshops can provide hands-on experience and clarify any lingering doubts. By broadening your sources and seeking expert advice, you can refine your identification skills and increase your confidence in recognizing medicinal plants accurately.

Warm Belly Massage Oil Elixir for Cramps

This warming, pain-relieving oil is formulated to provide calming cramp relief.

Ingredients:

½ cup Jojoba oil or coconut oil (carrier oil)

10 drops Clary Sage essential oil – relaxes the uterus and balances hormones

10 drops Lavender essential oil – calms nerves and reduces bloating

10 drops Peppermint essential oil – relieves tension and cools inflammation

Instructions:

Mix oils in a small glass bottle.

Massage onto the abdomen and lower back as needed.

Environmental factors can also play a significant role in plant misidentification. Seasonal variations, for instance, affect leaf color, with autumn bringing a tapestry of hues that can obscure the usual green identifiers. A plant easily recognized in spring might appear entirely different as it prepares for winter. Similarly, drought conditions can stunt growth, making a species appear smaller or less vibrant than expected. These changes can deceive even the most attentive gardener, leading to confusion and errors. Understanding these environmental influences allows you to anticipate and account for such variations, adapting your identification approach as needed.

Collaborating with peers is another effective strategy for enhancing accuracy in plant identification. Participating in group foraging expeditions fosters a learning community where individuals can share experiences and knowledge, discuss observations, and collectively verify plant characteristics. Engaging in online plant identification forums provides an additional platform for exchanging information and seeking guidance from a diverse audience. These interactions expand your understanding and reinforce your learning through shared experiences and collective wisdom. By working together, you can build a support network that enriches your apothecary practice and enhances your botanical knowledge.

Burdock Root Mud Bath Elixir

A deeply purifying and skin-rejuvenating mud bath elixir infused with burdock root to support detoxification, skin health, and relaxation.

Ingredients:

½ cup burdock root, dried and finely ground (for detoxification and skin purification)

1 cup bentonite clay or Rhassoul clay (to draw out toxins and remineralize the skin). Rhassoul clay has a higher silica and magnesium content.

½ cup Epsom salt (for muscle relaxation and magnesium replenishment)

½ teaspoon ginger powder (for circulation and anti-inflammatory benefits)

1 tablespoon raw honey (for hydration and antimicrobial properties)

5 drops of lavender essential oil (optional for calming effects)

5 drops of rosemary essential oil (optional for circulation support)

Warm water or herbal tea infusion (to achieve desired consistency)

Instructions:

Mix burdock root powder, bentonite clay, Epsom salt, and ginger powder in a bowl until well combined.

Slowly add warm water or an herbal tea infusion (such as chamomile or nettle tea) until a smooth, mud-like consistency is formed.

Stir in raw honey and essential oils if using.

Fill a bathtub with warm water and apply the mud elixir to the body, allowing it to dry for 10–15 minutes before soaking in the tub.

Soak for 20–30 minutes, massaging the skin gently to exfoliate before rinsing with warm water.

Follow with a moisturizing oil such as jojoba or almond oil to lock in hydration.

Benefits:

- ✔ *Detoxifies & Deeply Cleanses – Burdock root and clay help remove impurities and support skin health.*
- ✔ *Improves Circulation & Relieves Inflammation – Ginger and rosemary promote blood flow and muscle relaxation.*
- ✔ *Nourishes & Hydrates – Honey provides deep skin hydration and antimicrobial protection.*
- ✔ *Replenishes Essential Minerals – Epsom salt restores magnesium for muscle recovery and relaxation.*

As you navigate the intricacies of plant identification, it's essential to approach each encounter with a spirit of curiosity and a willingness to learn from mistakes. Every misstep offers an opportunity for growth, refining your skills, and deepening your connection to the plants you study. With patience and persistence, you will develop a keen eye for detail, an understanding of environmental influences, and a network of resources to support your efforts. This chapter has equipped you with strategies to address common identification challenges, empowering you to accurately recognize the plants that form the foundation of your home apothecary.

By integrating these troubleshooting techniques into your practice, you ensure the integrity and safety of your herbal remedies. As you expand your knowledge, you'll find that each new plant becomes a familiar friend, its unique traits etched into your memory. With this solid foundation in plant identification, you are now ready to explore the next chapter, where we delve into the fascinating world of adaptogens, uncovering their unique benefits and how they can enhance your beauty, health, and well-being.

Chapter Four

Exploring the World of Adaptogens

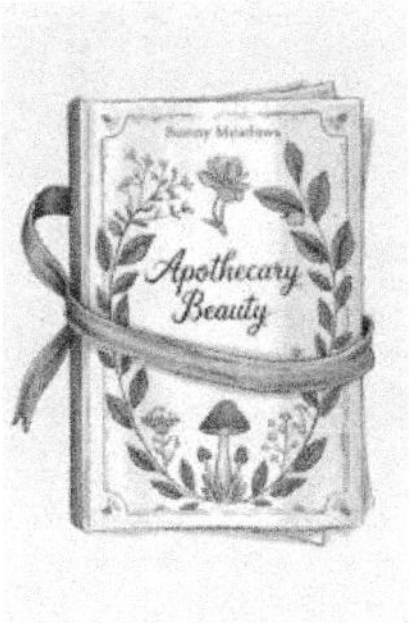

Adaptogens are renowned for their remarkable ability to help the body navigate the stresses of life. Their name derives from the word "adapt," reflecting their unique role in helping you adjust to various physical and mental stressors. These remarkable plants and mushrooms naturally balance the body's response to stress, enhancing resilience and vitality without the side effects often associated with synthetic solutions.

Adaptogens interact with the body's stress-response system, specifically the hypothalamus-pituitary-adrenal (HPA) axis, which regulates how your body reacts to stress. When faced with stressors, this system is activated to release hormones like cortisol, which prepare the body to cope. However, chronic stress can lead to an overactive HPA axis, resulting in a range of health issues such as fatigue, anxiety, and weakened immunity. Adaptogens intervene by modulating the HPA axis, helping normalize hormone levels and promoting homeostasis—a state of equilibrium in the body. This balancing act sets adaptogens apart, supporting your body's ability to cope with stress and maintain stability, even in challenging circumstances.

Lion's Mane Brain Boost Latte

Enhances focus, memory, and mental clarity—great as a morning coffee alternative.

1 cup warm oat or coconut milk

½ tsp lion's mane mushroom powder

1 tsp raw cacao powder

½ tsp cinnamon

1 tsp maple syrup

Optional: ¼ tsp vanilla extract

Blend for a frothy texture.

The benefits of adaptogens extend beyond stress management. By supporting the body's adaptive responses, these plants enhance overall resilience. They bolster your energy levels, improve endurance, and fortify your immune system, making you less susceptible to illness. For instance, Asian ginseng, a well-known adaptogen, is celebrated for boosting stamina and cognitive function. This makes it a popular choice among those seeking to improve their mental and physical performance. Similarly, rhodiola, a plant native to the cold regions of Europe and Asia, has been used for centuries to battle fatigue and enhance mental clarity. Its adaptogenic properties help you stay sharp and focused, even under pressure.

Goji Berry & Hibiscus Beauty Tonic

Packed with antioxidants to support glowing skin and hydration.

1 cup brewed hibiscus tea

1 tbsp dried goji berries (steeped in tea)

½ tsp honey or coconut nectar

Splash of lemon juice

Ice cubes for a refreshing version

Incorporating adaptogens into your daily routine is a powerful way to support your well-being. These herbs can be consumed in various forms, including teas, tinctures, mocktails, and capsules, offering flexibility in integrating them into your lifestyle. Many enjoy starting their day with a cup of adaptogenic tea, such as ashwagandha or holy basil, to promote calmness and focus. Adaptogen tinctures may be added to smoothies or juices for a convenient boost of resilience on the go. However, it's important to remember that while adaptogens offer temporary support, they are not a panacea for long-term stress. It is essential to address the root causes of stress through mindfulness, lifestyle changes, and self-care practices.

Lavender & Holy Basil Stress-Relief Tea

A floral, calming tea that soothes anxiety and uplifts the mood.

1 cup hot water

1 tsp dried tulsi (holy basil)

½ tsp dried lavender

½ tsp chamomile (optional)

1 tsp honey

Optional: splash of almond or oat milk for creaminess

Steep for 10 minutes, strain, and enjoy.

Before introducing adaptogens to your regimen, consider consulting a healthcare provider, especially if you have underlying health conditions or take medications. Although adaptogens are generally safe, they can interact with certain medications and conditions, such as hypertension or diabetes. Your holistic healthcare provider can help you determine the appropriate adaptogens and dosages for your needs, ensuring you gain the maximum benefit without unintended side effects. As with any herbal supplement, it's always wise to start with a low dose and gradually increase it as your body acclimates. This cautious approach allows you to monitor how your body responds and make any necessary adjustments.

Mucuna Pruriens Bliss Elixir

Promotes dopamine production, mood balance, and relaxation.

1 cup warm almond or coconut milk

½ tsp mucuna pruriens (velvet bean or cowage) powder

1 tsp cacao powder

½ tsp cinnamon

1 tsp maple syrup

Blend for a creamy, mood-boosting drink.

The beauty of adaptogens lies in their versatility and gentle nature. Unlike many pharmaceutical interventions, adaptogens are nontoxic in regular doses, making them a safe option for most people. Their ability to support the body without overwhelming it aligns with the principles of holistic wellness, where the focus is on nurturing and enhancing your body's natural functions. By incorporating adaptogens into your lifestyle, you embrace a proactive approach to health that empowers you to take charge of your well-being and cultivate a sense of balance in both body and mind. This chapter invites you to explore the fascinating world of adaptogens, unlocking their potential to transform your body with health and enhanced vitality.

Visual Element: Adaptogen Identification Guide

To help you recognize adaptogens, consider creating a visual guide that includes images and descriptions of common adaptogenic plants. This guide can serve as a valuable reference, helping you identify these plants and mushrooms in your garden or local area. Include details such as leaf shape, flower characteristics, and preferred growing conditions, ensuring you have the information to cultivate and harvest these powerful allies in your quest for balance and resilience.

The Science of Adaptogens: Emerging Research & Modern Insights

Scientific exploration has taken a keen interest in adaptogens, revealing new insights that blend traditional knowledge with modern research. Among the most intriguing areas of study is the role of adaptogens in combating neuroinflammation and promoting cognitive function. A 2023 mini-review has highlighted the remarkable effects of compounds such as curcumin, resveratrol, and ginsenosides. These substances have shown promise in reducing neuroinflammation, a key factor in neurodegenerative diseases like Alzheimer's and Parkinson's. Curcumin, a polyphenol derived from the turmeric plant, has been particularly noted for its ability to cross the blood-brain barrier, offering neuroprotective properties that may help safeguard against the progressive deterioration of neurons. In the garden, turmeric's bright orange rhizomes are a testament to its potent potential, bridging the gap between natural remedies and cutting-edge science.

Ashwagandha Rose Almond Milk

A nourishing, stress-relieving, and heart-opening blend.

1 cup warm almond milk

½ tsp ashwagandha powder

1 tsp dried rose petals (or ½ tsp rose water)

1 tsp honey

¼ tsp cardamom powder

Optional: Blend with ½ tsp ghee for extra nourishment

The stress-relieving qualities of adaptogens have long been celebrated, and recent studies continue to underscore their importance for mental health. In South America, Maca root (an adaptogenic herb) was used in ritual drinks that promoted stamina and stress resilience. Adaptogens like ashwagandha and rhodiola are gaining recognition for their ability to alleviate symptoms of stress and improve mood. Ashwagandha, often referred to as Indian ginseng, has been used for centuries in Ayurvedic medicine to promote balance and reduce anxiety. It was usually prepared as a tonic to unwind in the evening, much like modern adaptogenic nightcaps. Modern research supports these traditional claims; studies suggest that ashwagandha supplementation can significantly reduce anxiety and depression symptoms by moderating cortisol levels, a primary stress hormone. Rhodiola enhances mental endurance and reduces fatigue, providing a complementary approach. Its unique compounds, such as rosavin and salidroside, have been found to improve cognitive function and mitigate stress-related fatigue, making it a valuable ally in today's fast-paced world. Ginseng and Rhodiola rosea were used by scholars, monks, and warriors to help the body resist fatigue and enhance endurance without overstimulating. Together, these adaptogens provide a natural means of stress reduction, allowing you to navigate life's challenges with greater ease and resilience.

Eleuthero & Ginseng Energy Tea

A natural energy booster without the crash of caffeine.

1 cup hot water

1 tsp dried eleuthero root (steep for 10 minutes)

½ tsp ginseng root (optional)

½ tsp honey

Optional: splash of lemon juice for freshness

The immune-boosting properties of adaptogens are another area of growing interest. Reishi mushrooms, often called the "mushroom of immortality," are being studied for their potential to enhance immune response and offer anti-cancer benefits. These fungi contain polysaccharides and triterpenoids, compounds known to support the immune system by increasing the activity of white blood cells. In traditional Chinese medicine, reishi has been used to fortify vitality and longevity, and modern science is beginning to validate these age-old practices. Emperors and monks used reishi to promote tranquility and spiritual clarity—a function similar to alcohol in social or ceremonial settings but without intoxication. Incorporating reishi into your herbal repertoire can provide a gentle yet effective way to bolster your body's natural defenses, helping you maintain health and well-being throughout the seasons.

Reishi Hot Cocoa

A rich, chocolatey drink that calms the mind and supports immunity.

1 cup oat or almond milk

1 tbsp raw cacao powder

½ tsp reishi mushroom powder

1 tsp maple syrup

¼ tsp cinnamon

Optional: a pinch of cayenne for a spicy kick

In the realm of weight management and metabolic health, adaptogens are offering new possibilities. Compounds like salidroside, found in Rhodiola, have been investigated for their role in regulating body weight and metabolism. Animal studies indicate that salidroside can decrease food intake and body weight while improving glucose and insulin tolerance. These findings suggest potential applications for adaptogens in managing metabolic disorders, providing a natural alternative to conventional treatments. Adaptogens like Rhodiola can contribute to overall vitality by supporting metabolic health, enhancing energy levels, and promoting a more balanced lifestyle.

Rhodiola Brain-Boosting Tea (For Focus & Memory)

A natural energy booster without the crash of caffeine for studying, working, or before an important task.

1 cup hot water

1 tsp dried Rhodiola root

1 tsp Ginkgo Biloba (improves circulation and cognitive function)

½ tsp Dried Peppermint – cooling and supports focus

Steep for 10 minutes

Optional: 1 tsp raw honey

Interestingly, the benefits of adaptogens extend beyond internal health, with recent research exploring their impact on hair growth. Ginseng, a well-known adaptogen, is being studied for its capacity to promote hair health. Red ginseng extract has been shown to stimulate hair follicles and improve blood circulation to the scalp, potentially enhancing hair growth. This discovery opens new avenues for using adaptogens in natural beauty regimens, offering a holistic approach to hair care that aligns with the broader principles of wellness and self-care. As you cultivate ginseng in your garden, its roots hold the promise of supporting your internal health and enriching your external appearance.

Red Ginseng Hair Growth Drink (Warm or Iced)

Red Ginseng boosts blood flow to hair follicles and modulates stress hormones, which can help with stress-related hair loss.

1 cup hot water

1 tsp red ginseng powder (or 1 red ginseng root, simmered for 15–20 minutes)

1 tsp raw honey (or maple syrup)

½ tsp fresh grated ginger (optional for circulation)

Splash of lemon juice (for taste and vitamin C)

Optional: 1 tsp collagen powder (for extra hair growth support)

Advances in herbal medicine often highlight the synergistic effects of combining different adaptogens and supplements. Recent studies have proposed that combining adaptogens like ashwagandha with other supplements, such as magnesium, may improve sleep quality and mental health. This combination leverages the calming effects of ashwagandha with magnesium's muscle-relaxing properties, offering a comprehensive approach to managing stress, enhancing relaxation, and alleviating symptoms of anxiety and insomnia. These findings underscore the potential for integrative therapies that draw on the strengths of multiple natural remedies, creating personalized solutions that address individual needs.

Lemon Balm & Passionflower Sleep Tonic

A soothing nighttime drink that calms the nervous system and promotes deep sleep.

1 cup hot water

1 tsp dried lemon balm

1 tsp dried passionflower

½ tsp chamomile flowers (optional)

1 tsp honey or agave

Optional: splash of tart cherry juice (natural source of melatonin)

Steep herbs for 10 minutes, strain, and sip before bed.

The evolving landscape of adaptogen research offers an exciting glimpse into the future of herbal medicine. As scientists continue to explore these remarkable plants, they uncover new layers of understanding that can inform and enhance your apothecary practices. By staying attuned to these developments, you can integrate the latest insights into your health regimen, maximizing the benefits of adaptogens in your daily life. The garden becomes a place of beauty and a living laboratory where tradition and innovation coexist, offering endless possibilities for growth and discovery.

Using Adaptogen Drinks as Alcohol Alternatives

Long before the wellness industry began branding "functional beverages," adaptogenic herbs and mushrooms were used in traditional medicine systems for stress relief, relaxation, and even social bonding. In Siberia and Central Asia, Rhodiola and Eleuthero (Siberian ginseng) were brewed into warming tonics to protect against harsh environments and mental fatigue, sometimes replacing alcohol in ceremonies.

Rhodiola Berry Cooler

A fruity, adaptogen-rich mocktail that provides a mental energy and mood-balancing boost.

1 cup hibiscus or berry tea, chilled

½ tsp Rhodiola powder

1 tsp honey

½ cup sparkling water

Fresh berries and mint for garnish

Traditional Chinese used Schisandra berry to increase vitality and relieve stress while enhancing mental focus, an effect reminiscent of specific "euphoric" alcohol alternatives today.

Schisandra Berry Elixir

Supports liver health, mental clarity, and adrenal balance.

1 cup brewed Schisandra berry tea (steep 1 tbsp dried berries for 15 minutes)

½ tsp fresh ginger juice

½ tsp honey or coconut nectar

Splash of lemon juice

Ice cubes (optional)

The concept of Rasayana (rejuvenation) in Ayurveda emphasizes herbs that promote longevity, reduce stress, and restore balance to the mind and body. Holy Basil (Tulsi) was considered a sacred herb that protected against stress and illness. It was commonly consumed in tea or elixirs to promote mental clarity and relaxation.

Sparkling Tulsi-Lavender Lemonade

A refreshing, floral drink that supports the nervous system and digestion.

1 cup brewed and cooled tulsi (holy basil) tea

½ cup sparkling water

1 tsp fresh lemon juice

½ tsp lavender honey (or regular honey)

Ice cubes

The adverse effects of alcohol (hangovers, dehydration, premature aging, addiction risks, inflammation) are now widely understood, leading to a cultural reevaluation of drinking habits. Adaptogens offer relaxation without intoxication, making them appealing to those seeking healthier ways to unwind. Adaptogens and alcohol have almost opposite effects on the body. While alcohol is a depressant that can impair cognitive function, disrupt sleep, and contribute to stress eventually, adaptogens are natural substances that help the body resist stress and restore balance.

Maca Chai Latte

Great for energy balance and hormone support.

1 cup brewed chai tea

1 tsp maca powder

½ cup frothed almond or coconut milk

1 tsp honey

Pinch of nutmeg

The launch of Kin Euphorics, Three Spirit, and De Soi brought adaptogenic elixirs into mainstream culture. Wellness influencers, celebrities, and functional beverage startups have normalized "social tonics" as alcohol replacements, featuring ingredients like Ashwagandha, Holy Basil, and Reishi. The rapid expansion of adaptogen bars, mocktail lounges, and wellness cafes offers botanical-based alternatives to traditional cocktails.

Kava Coconut Cooler

A relaxing alternative to alcohol, traditionally used for stress relief and social relaxation.

1 cup brewed kava root tea (steep kava powder in warm—not boiling—water for 15 minutes)

½ cup coconut milk

1 tsp honey or coconut sugar

Pinch of cinnamon

Ice cubes for a chilled version

People are increasingly interested in longevity, stress management, and mental clarity—all things that alcohol harms but adaptogens support. Health-conscious individuals are replacing alcohol with adaptogens for better sleep, mood balance, and cognitive function. The idea of "social drinking" without alcohol is growing, and adaptogenic drinks offer a ritualistic experience similar to cocktails. Unlike traditional soft drinks or plain water, adaptogenic beverages provide physiological benefits that enhance well-being, reinforcing the shift away from alcohol.

Golden Moon Milk (Ashwagandha & Turmeric)

A warm, creamy drink that soothes stress and promotes restful sleep.

1 cup warm milk (dairy or plant-based)

½ tsp ashwagandha powder

½ tsp turmeric

¼ tsp cinnamon

1 tsp honey or maple syrup

Pinch of black pepper (enhances turmeric absorption)

Optional: ½ tsp ghee or coconut oil

The use of adaptogens in place of alcohol is part of a more extensive cultural transformation that prioritizes holistic health, mental clarity, and sustainability. Ancient herbal traditions have evolved into a modern movement, reshaping social drinking habits. From monks sipping Reishi for spiritual clarity to sober, curious millennials toasting ashwagandha mocktails, the journey of adaptogens replacing alcohol is deeply rooted in history and driven by modern innovation. As the market continues to grow, expect more sophisticated adaptogenic drinks, alcohol-free cocktail bars, and social rituals centered around feeling good—without the booze.

Chaga Vanilla Latte

An earthy, coffee alternative with immune-boosting and stress-reducing properties.

1 cup brewed Chaga mushroom tea (steep Chaga chunks or powder for 20+ minutes)

½ cup warm oat or coconut milk

1 tsp vanilla extract

1 tsp maple syrup

½ tsp cinnamon

Optional: blend with ½ tsp coconut oil for creaminess

Adaptogens reveal more about their potential to support health and well-being with each new study. These insights resonate with the broader themes of sustainability and self-sufficiency, as they empower you to make informed choices about your health. As you explore the world of adaptogens, you'll find that these plants offer a unique blend of ancient wisdom and modern science, providing tools to cultivate resilience and vitality in your life. The next chapter will delve deeper into crafting remedies for everyday ailments, building on the knowledge and skills you've gathered to create a comprehensive apothecary that supports your holistic wellness journey.

Chapter Five

Crafting Remedies for Everyday Ailments

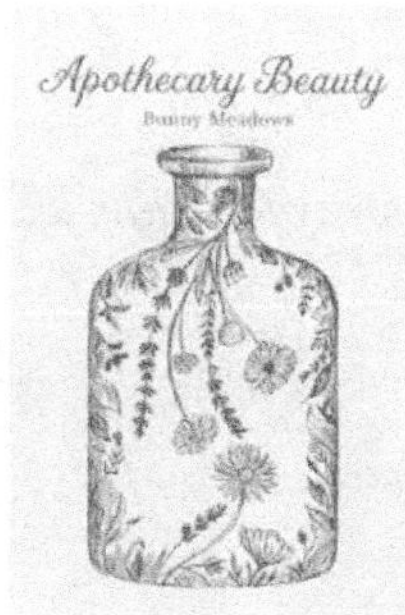

Jasmine produces fragrant white flowers that bloom at night, releasing a sweet, intoxicating scent. It's perfect for an evening garden or balcony. In this chapter, we explore the art of crafting quick remedies for stress and anxiety, harnessing the calming effects of these cherished herbs to restore balance and peace to your life.

Hibiscus Face Toner Elixir

A rejuvenating, antioxidant-rich facial toner that brightens the skin, tightens pores and promotes a radiant complexion.

Ingredients:

½ cup dried hibiscus flowers (rich in natural AHAs and antioxidants)

1 cup rose water or distilled water (for hydration and toning)

1 tablespoon witch hazel (for pore tightening and oil control)

½ teaspoon raw apple cider vinegar (optional, for pH balance)

5 drops rosehip seed oil (for anti-aging and hydration)

3–5 drops of lavender essential oil (soothing and antimicrobial)

Instructions:

Brew Hibiscus Tea: Steep hibiscus flowers in 1 cup of hot water for 10–15 minutes, then strain and let cool completely.

Mix Ingredients: In a glass bottle, combine hibiscus tea, rose water, witch hazel, apple cider vinegar, rosehip oil, and lavender essential oil.

Shake well before each use.

Apply with a cotton pad or spritz onto clean skin as a refreshing facial mist.

Benefits:

- ✔ *Brightens Skin & Reduces Dark Spots – Hibiscus is high in vitamin C and natural exfoliants.*
- ✔ *Tightens Pores & Controls Oil – Witch hazel and rose water tone and balance the skin.*
- ✔ *Promotes Hydration & Anti-Aging – Rosehip oil supports collagen production.*
- ✔ *Soothes & Reduces Inflammation – Lavender and hibiscus calm redness and irritation.*

Chamomile, with its delicate, daisy-like flowers, has been celebrated for centuries as a natural remedy for relaxation and inflammation. This gentle herb works by interacting with the nervous system, promoting a sense of calm and easing tension. Its anti-inflammatory properties also extend to the body, soothing aches and discomfort. Lavender, known for its fragrant purple blooms, enhances mood by interacting with neurotransmitters that regulate emotional well-being. Together, these herbs create a powerful duo, offering a holistic approach to stress relief that nurtures mind and body. The calming aroma of chamomile and lavender has long been revered for its ability to ease the mind and body, offering a natural respite from the stresses of daily life. Often overlooked in the bustle of modern living, these humble plants can transform your evenings into moments of tranquility.

Lavender Bath Salt Scrub

A calming, exfoliating scrub that soothes the skin, relaxes the body and uplifts the senses—perfect for unwinding and restoring balance.

Ingredients:

1 cup Epsom salt (rich in magnesium to relax muscles)

½ cup sea salt or Himalayan pink salt (detoxifying and mineral-rich)

¼ cup carrier oil (e.g., sweet almond, jojoba, or coconut oil)

2 tablespoons dried lavender flowers (gentle exfoliation and calming aroma)

10–15 drops of lavender essential oil (promotes relaxation and skin healing)

1 tablespoon raw honey (optional for moisture and antibacterial benefits)

Instructions:

Combine Epsom salt, sea salt, and dried lavender in a bowl.

Stir in the carrier oil until the mixture resembles wet sand.

Add lavender essential oil and honey (if using), mixing thoroughly.

Store in a glass jar with a lid.

To Use:

Massage onto damp skin in circular motions while in the bath or shower.

Let the scrub sit on the skin for a minute or two to absorb its benefits.

Rinse with warm water and pat dry.

Benefits:

✔ *Gently Exfoliates & Softens Skin – Salts and lavender remove dead skin cells.*

- ✔ *Relaxes Muscles & Nerves – Epsom salt and lavender calm the body and mind.*
- ✔ *Hydrates & Nourishes – Carrier oil and honey leave the skin supple and moisturized.*
- ✔ *Uplifts Mood & Promotes Sleep – Lavender aroma reduces stress and promotes restful sleep.*

One of the simplest ways to enjoy the benefits of chamomile and lavender is through a soothing tea blend. To prepare this calming infusion, combine equal parts dried chamomile and lavender flowers in a teapot. Pour boiling water over the herbs and steep for five to ten minutes, allowing the flavors and benefits to meld. Strain the liquid and savor the delicate aroma as you sip, letting each warm cup wash away the day's worries. For a luxurious bath experience, consider crafting herbal stress relief bath salts. Combine Epsom salts with a few drops of chamomile and lavender essential oils, then sprinkle them into a warm bath. As you soak, the calming scents envelop you, melting tension and soothing sore muscles.

Castor Oil Wrap for Sore Muscles & Inflammation Relief

A deeply penetrating, anti-inflammatory remedy using castor oil to soothe sore muscles, reduce tension, and promote circulation.

Ingredients:

¼ cup organic castor oil (deeply moisturizing and anti-inflammatory)

1 soft cotton or flannel cloth (large enough to cover the sore area)

1 hot water bottle or heating pad (for enhanced absorption)

1 sheet of plastic wrap or wax paper (to prevent mess)

5 drops peppermint essential oil (optional, for cooling pain relief)

5 drops of ginger essential oil (optional for warming and circulation)

Instructions:

Prepare the Wrap:

Soak the cotton or flannel cloth in castor oil, ensuring it is well-saturated but not dripping.

Add peppermint and ginger essential oils to the oil before applying.

Apply to Sore Muscles:

Place the castor oil-soaked cloth over the sore area (back, shoulders, knees, or other affected area).

Cover with plastic wrap or wax paper to keep the oil from staining fabrics.

Apply Heat:

Place a heating pad or hot water bottle over the wrap.

Leave for 20–45 minutes, allowing the oil to penetrate deeply.

Clean Up & Rest:

Remove the wrap and gently wipe off excess oil with a warm cloth.

Relax and allow the healing effects to continue.

Benefits:

- ✔ *Reduces Muscle Soreness & Tension – Castor oil profoundly penetrates to ease inflammation.*
- ✔ *Boosts Circulation & Detoxification – Warming oils and heat promote blood flow.*
- ✔ *Soothes Nerve Pain & Joint Stiffness – Helps with chronic pain and recovery.*
- ✔ *Hydrates & Nourishes Skin – Castor oil provides deep moisture while aiding healing.*

Pain relief herbal soaks and compresses offer another avenue for relaxation. To create a compress, steep a handful of chamomile flowers in hot water until the liquid is fragrant, then soak a cloth in the infusion, wring out the excess, and apply it to areas of tension, such as the neck or shoulders. The warmth and herbal properties work in tandem to ease discomfort and promote relaxation, providing a simple yet effective remedy for stress-induced muscle aches. These remedies offer immediate relief and create a comforting ritual that can become a cherished part of your self-care routine.

Pain Relief Salve

This soothing, anti-inflammatory herbal salve is designed to ease muscle pain, joint discomfort, and minor aches.

Ingredients:

½ cup olive oil or coconut oil (for a nourishing base)

¼ cup beeswax (for a smooth, firm texture)

2 tablespoons arnica flowers (reduces muscle soreness and inflammation)

2 tablespoons St. John's Wort (helps with nerve pain and healing)

1 tablespoon cayenne pepper (natural pain reliever that increases circulation)

1 tablespoon ginger powder or freshly grated ginger (anti-inflammatory and warming)

10 drops peppermint essential oil (cooling relief and muscle relaxation)

10 drops eucalyptus essential oil (soothes tension and promotes blood flow)

5 drops lavender essential oil (calming and supports healing)

Instructions:

Infuse the Oil:

Warm the olive oil with arnica, St. John's Wort, cayenne, and ginger in a double boiler or a heat-safe jar over low heat.

Let it infuse for 30-60 minutes, stirring occasionally.

Strain out the herbs using cheesecloth or a fine strainer.

Prepare the Salve:

Melt the beeswax in the infused oil over low heat.

Remove from heat and stir in essential oils.

Store & Use:

Pour into a small glass jar or tin and let cool until solid.

Apply to sore muscles, joints, or tension areas as needed.

Benefits:

- ✔ *Reduces Inflammation & Soreness – Arnica and ginger soothe muscle pain.*
- ✔ *Boosts Circulation & Eases Joint Pain – Cayenne and peppermint improve blood flow.*
- ✔ *Soothes Nerve Pain & Tension – St. John's Wort and eucalyptus calm the nervous system.*
- ✔ *Provides Cooling & Warming Relief – A balanced effect to relax tight areas.*

The science behind herbal stress relief is rooted in the herbs' ability to interact with the body's stress-response system. Chamomile and lavender influence neurotransmitters and hormones, such as cortisol, which affect stress and anxiety. By modulating these chemicals, the herbs help stabilize mood and reduce the physiological effects of stress. Research supports these benefits; a study published in 2022 found that inhalation of aromatherapy with lavender and chamomile essential oils significantly decreased levels of depression, anxiety, and stress in older adults (Source 1). This evidence underscores the potential of these herbs to promote mental and emotional well-being.

~

Hypericum Mood-Boosting Elixir

A natural remedy for stress, anxiety, mild depression, and nervous system balance.

Ingredients:

1 tablespoon dried hypericum flowers (or two tablespoons fresh)

1 cup warm water (not boiling, to preserve medicinal compounds)

½ teaspoon raw honey (optional for calming effects)

½ teaspoon fresh lemon juice (for vitamin C and detox support)

¼ teaspoon cinnamon (optional for circulation and warmth)

Instructions:

Steep hypericum flowers in warm water for 10–15 minutes.

Strain and stir in honey, lemon juice, and cinnamon.

Enjoy warm as a calming and mood-supporting herbal tea.

Benefits:

✔ *Supports nervous system health*

✔ *Reduces stress and mild anxiety*

✔ *Balances mood*

~

Integrating these remedies into your daily life can be both simple and rewarding. Establishing an evening herbal tea ritual provides a moment of calm at the end of each day, setting the stage for restful sleep. Consider incorporating aromatherapy with essential oils into your routine; a few drops of lavender oil on your pillow or in a diffuser can create a serene atmosphere conducive to relaxation. For those experiencing muscle soreness, an anti-inflammatory arnica salve offers targeted relief. Gently massage the salve onto affected areas to reduce inflammation and discomfort, allowing you to unwind with ease.

Interactive Element: Evening Herbal Tea or Mocktail Ritual

Create a personalized evening tea ritual by selecting your favorite calming herbs, such as chamomile and lavender. Designate a special teacup or mug for this ritual, and set aside time each evening to prepare your tea. As you sip, focus on the warmth of the cup in your hands and the soothing aroma of the herbs. Reflect on the day's events, and let any tension melt away with each sip. This mindful practice enhances the benefits of the herbs and cultivates a sense of peace and presence, grounding you in the moment and preparing you for a restful night's sleep.

Herbal Solutions for Digestive Health

In the quiet moments of tending to your garden, the familiar scents of peppermint and ginger may greet you, each carrying a promise of relief from digestive discomforts. These herbs are not just culinary delights but powerful allies in promoting digestive wellness. Peppermint, with its cool menthol aroma, is renowned for its ability to soothe the stomach. It relaxes the gastrointestinal tract muscles, easing symptoms such as gas, bloating, and indigestion. This relaxing effect makes peppermint a cornerstone in natural digestive health, offering comfort when your stomach feels unsettled.

Morning: Peppermint Gut-Healing Elixir

Start the day with a gentle digestive boost to soothe the gut and support digestion by repairing the gut lining and relieving bloating.

Ingredients:

1 cup Warm Peppermint Tea – relaxes the digestive tract, reduces bloating

½ tsp Ginger Juice or Powder – stimulates digestion and relieves gas

½ tsp Slippery Elm Powder – coats the gut lining and reduces irritation

1 tbsp Aloe Vera Juice – heals and soothes the gut

½ tbsp Apple Cider Vinegar (with the mother) – aids digestion (optional)

1 tsp Raw Honey – prebiotic support for gut flora

Instructions:

Brew peppermint tea and let it cool slightly.

Add ginger, slippery elm, aloe vera juice, and honey.

Stir well and drink on an empty stomach.

Meanwhile, ginger, with its warm and spicy bite, aids digestion by stimulating digestive enzymes. These enzymes are critical in breaking down food, ensuring a smoother digestive process. Ginger's anti-inflammatory properties also reduce nausea and support overall gut health, making it a versatile addition to your herbal toolkit.

How to Make Ginger & Lemongrass Tea

Ingredients:

1-inch piece of fresh ginger, sliced

2-3 fresh or dried lemongrass stalks, chopped

2 cups of water

Optional: *raw honey and lemon for extra flavor*

Instructions:

Bring water to a boil, then add ginger and lemongrass.

Simmer for 10-15 minutes.

Strain and enjoy warm.

To harness the benefits of these herbs, consider incorporating them into simple, effective recipes that support digestive health. A ginger and turmeric digestive tonic is a potent blend that combines the anti-inflammatory power of turmeric with the digestive stimulation of ginger. To prepare, simmer fresh ginger slices in water with a dash of turmeric powder; add honey for sweetness if desired. This tonic not only aids digestion but also provides an anti-inflammatory boost, making it perfect for regular consumption. Another option is a peppermint and fennel seed chewable, which combines the soothing effects of peppermint with the gentle digestive support of fennel. These can be made by grinding the seeds and mixing them with a bit of honey to form small, chewable balls. Both recipes are designed to be easy to prepare and integrate into your daily routine, providing natural relief without synthetic alternatives.

Probiotic Shot

A quick gut-friendly probiotic shot that maintains healthy digestion and balances gut bacteria.

Ingredients:

½ cup Coconut Water, Kefir, or Kombucha – rich in probiotics

1 tsp Lemon Juice – alkalizes the gut and supports digestion

½ tsp Ginger Powder – aids digestion and reduces bloating

Instructions:

Mix ingredients in a glass.

Drink before meals to support digestion and prevent bloating.

Benefits:

✔ *Boosts gut-friendly bacteria and*

✔ *Enhances nutrient absorption*

The efficacy of these herbs lies in their ability to support the digestive system's natural processes. Peppermint's menthol content relaxes gastrointestinal muscles and has an antispasmodic effect, reducing cramps and discomfort. Meanwhile, ginger's role in stimulating saliva and bile production enhances the breakdown of food, facilitating better nutrient absorption. These properties make ginger particularly beneficial before meals, preparing the digestive system for the task ahead. A cup of ginger tea about 20–30 minutes before eating can prime your body for optimal digestion. For peppermint tea, one to two cups daily, especially after meals, can help maintain digestive health and alleviate symptoms of indigestion. It's important to adjust the dosage based on sensitivity and personal response, as peppermint can sometimes exacerbate conditions like acid reflux in susceptible individuals.

Gut-Healing Peppermint Smoothie

This nutrient-rich smoothie is packed with prebiotics, probiotics, and anti-inflammatory herbs.

Ingredients:

1 cup Coconut Yogurt or Almond Milk – probiotic support

½ cup Fresh Cucumber – hydrating and cooling for the gut

1 tbsp Ground Flaxseeds or Chia Seeds – prebiotic fiber

½ tsp Fresh Mint Leaves or Peppermint Extract – supports digestion

½ tsp Turmeric Powder – reduces gut inflammation

1 tsp Raw Honey or Maple Syrup – nourishes gut bacteria

Instructions:

Blend all ingredients until smooth.

Enjoy as a light meal or post-lunch digestive support.

Benefits:

✔ *Provides gut-friendly fiber, probiotics, and cooling digestion support.*

Neem (Azadirachta indica) is a powerful medicinal herb with antibacterial, antifungal, anti-inflammatory, and detoxifying properties that make it excellent for gut health. It helps balance the gut microbiome, reduce bloating, and support digestion. Neem helps eliminate harmful pathogens like H. pylori, which can cause ulcers and acid reflux. It reduces harmful bacteria while preserving beneficial gut flora. Neem acts as a natural antiparasitic, clearing out worms and intestinal infections. Neem's strong anti-inflammatory properties help heal conditions like IBS, Crohn's, and colitis. Soothes irritation in the stomach lining and reduces acid reflux. Protects against leaky gut syndrome by reducing inflammation.

Probiotic-Enhanced Neem Gut Health Elixir

Probiotics and prebiotics elixir to support a healthy microbiome while detoxifying.

Ingredients:

½ tsp Neem powder – antibacterial and antifungal gut detox

1 tbsp Apple Cider Vinegar (with the mother) – boosts digestion and provides probiotics

1 tbsp Fresh Coconut Water or Kefir – introduces beneficial gut bacteria

½ tsp Ginger juice or powder – aids digestion and reduces bloating

½ tsp Flaxseed powder – provides prebiotic fiber for gut bacteria

½ tsp Turmeric powder – reduces inflammation and supports the microbiome

1 tsp Raw honey or Maple syrup – feeds good bacteria (optional)

½ cup Warm water – helps with absorption

Instructions:

Mix all ingredients in warm water (not too hot to preserve probiotics).

Stir well and drink on an empty stomach.

Wait at least 15 minutes before eating to allow absorption.

Benefits:

✔ *Repopulates healthy gut bacteria – balances microbiome*

✔ *Aids digestion & nutrient absorption – supports enzymes and stomach acid*

✔ *Supports detox & immunity – flushes toxins and strengthens gut lining*

✔ *Boosts energy & metabolism – promotes better digestion and gut balance*

Incorporating these herbal remedies into your lifestyle requires little more than a commitment to consistency and mindfulness. The process of brewing a cup of herbal tea or preparing a digestive tonic can become a ritual of care, a moment to pause and connect with the nurturing power of plants. As you develop a routine that includes these herbs, you support your digestive health and cultivate a deeper appreciation for the simple yet profound ways nature supports our well-being. With its abundance of healing plants, the garden becomes a source of empowerment, offering tools to enhance your health naturally and effectively.

Supporting Immunity with Natural Ingredients

In the midst of changing seasons, as the air turns crisp and the days grow shorter, the gentle rustle of leaves underfoot reminds us of the natural cycles that influence our well-being. Fortify your body against common colds and flu; certain herbs stand out as potent allies that support the immune system. Among these, echinacea and sage have been revered for their ability to bolster immunity. Echinacea, with its vibrant purple blooms, is more than just a garden beauty; Native Americans have traditionally used it for over 400 years to treat infections. Echinacea, known for its immune-boosting effects, is thought to enhance the body's resistance to illness, making it a valuable addition to your herbal repertoire. Sage offers antibacterial and antiviral properties, providing an extra layer of defense during the colder months. Together, these herbs form a formidable duo, ready to support your immune system's natural defenses.

Elderberry, with its deep purple berries and rich history in folk medicine, is another powerhouse for cold and flu prevention. This berry is rich in antioxidants and vitamins that boost the immune system. Its active compounds, such as anthocyanins, have been shown to reduce the severity and duration of cold and flu symptoms. Incorporating elderberry into your diet can be a proactive and delicious way to support your health as temperatures drop. A well-crafted echinacea and elderberry syrup can be a delightful addition to your daily regimen. To prepare, simmer elderberries with echinacea roots, a bit of honey, and a splash of lemon juice. This syrup tastes delightful and provides a powerful boost to your immune system. Another warming option is a herbal immune-supporting soup, where sage, garlic, and echinacea are simmered with nourishing vegetables to create a comforting dish that fortifies your defenses from the inside out.

Immunity-Boosting Herbal Elixir for Strength & Protection

This powerful immunity elixir is packed with antiviral, antibacterial, and adaptogenic herbs to help the body fight infections, reduce inflammation, and support overall immune health. Perfect for cold and flu prevention, recovery, and daily immune resilience.

Ingredients:

1 tbsp Dried Elderberries (or 2 tbsp fresh) – antiviral & immune-supporting

1 tbsp Astragalus Root (dried or fresh) – strengthens immune response

1 tbsp Fresh Ginger Root (chopped or ground) – antimicrobial and anti-inflammatory

½ tsp Turmeric Powder (or ½ tbsp Fresh Turmeric Root, ground) – supports immune and gut health

1 Cinnamon Stick (or ½ tsp ground Cinnamon) – warming and antimicrobial

1 Clove Garlic (optional, for extra strength) – antibacterial and antiviral

1 tbsp Raw Honey (or Maple Syrup for a vegan option) – soothes the throat and fights infection

1 tbsp Lemon Juice (freshly squeezed) – provides Vitamin C

2 cups filtered water

Instructions:

Step 1: *Grind the Herbs in the Mortar and Pestle*

Add elderberries, astragalus, ginger, turmeric, cinnamon, and garlic to the mortar.

Using the pestle, crush and grind them into a coarse paste. This releases their medicinal compounds for a more potent elixir.

Step 2: *Simmer and Extract the Herbal Goodness*

Transfer the ground mixture to a small pot.

Pour 2 cups of filtered water over the herbs.

Simmer on low heat for 20–30 minutes until reduced by half.

Strain using cheesecloth or a fine strainer into a clean glass jar.

Step 3: *Add Honey and Lemon*

Let the elixir cool slightly (not too hot, or it will destroy the honey's enzymes).

Stir in raw honey and fresh lemon juice.

Mix well and store in the fridge for up to 1 week.

How to Use:

✔ *Daily Immune Support: Take 1–2 tbsp daily (morning or afternoon).*

✔ *During Sickness: Take 1 tbsp every 3–4 hours to help recovery.*

✔ *As a Warm Tea: Mix 1 tbsp elixir in warm water for a soothing drink.*

Immunity Elixir Variations:

✔ *For a Spicy Kick: Add ¼ tsp cayenne pepper to boost circulation.*

✔ *For Extra Vitamin C: Add 1 tbsp rosehip powder for enhanced immune function.*

✔ *For Gut Health & Immunity: Add ½ tbsp apple cider vinegar for probiotic benefits.*

Final Tips for a Strong Immune System:

✔ *Stay hydrated – drink herbal teas and infused water.*

✔ *Get plenty of rest – immunity is strongest when well-rested.*

✔ *Eat whole, nutrient-rich foods – fresh fruits, veggies, and healthy fats.*

✔ *Manage stress – high cortisol weakens the immune system.*

~

Scientific studies lend credibility to the use of these herbs in supporting immunity. Clinical trials on echinacea have shown its potential to reduce the duration and severity of respiratory infections. One study found that echinacea may decrease the odds of developing a cold by 58% and shorten its duration by one to four days (Source 3). While results can vary, these findings underscore the herb's role as a supportive ally in maintaining health. Elderberry has also been the subject of numerous studies, with research suggesting that it can significantly reduce the severity and length of influenza symptoms when taken at the first sign of illness. These findings highlight the potential of elderberry to offer natural, practical support during flu season.

As the seasons shift, prepare your immune system for the challenges ahead. Embrace pre-winter herbal regimens to strengthen your defenses. Begin incorporating echinacea and elderberry into your routine well before the onset of the cold season. Regularly consume these herbs in teas, tinctures, or syrups to maintain a resilient immune system. During flu season, elderberry can serve as a frontline protector. A daily dose of elderberry syrup can provide continuous support, helping to ward off illness and keep you feeling vibrant and healthy. These practices, rooted in tradition and supported by science, offer a natural approach to nurturing your body's innate ability to fend off seasonal illnesses.

Skin Care from the Garden: Salves and Balms

The garden holds a treasure trove of herbs known for their remarkable skin-healing properties. Calendula, with its vivid orange petals, is celebrated for its ability to soothe inflammation and speed wound healing. It hydrates dry skin, offering a gentle touch for sensitive complexions. Aloe vera, known for its succulent leaves, provides deep hydration and cooling relief for burns and injuries. Chamomile, with its calming qualities, reduces redness and promotes skin repair, making it ideal for irritated skin. Yarrow, often overlooked, encourages circulation and tones the skin, aiding in wound healing with its subtle yet effective properties. Each of these herbs is vital in nurturing the skin, providing nourishment and protection from the elements.

Anti-Aging & Skin Rejuvenation Elixir Salve

A deeply nourishing salve to reduce wrinkles, improve skin elasticity, and hydrate dry skin. Perfect for fine lines, scars, sun damage, and dull skin.

Ingredients:

Rejuvenating Herbs (Choose 2–3 or mix all for extra potency)

2 tbsp Dried Rose Petals – (rich in antioxidants, help with skin elasticity)

2 tbsp Dried Hibiscus Flowers – (known as the "Botox plant," firm skin)

2 tbsp Dried Calendula Flowers – (speeds up skin healing and soothes inflammation)

2 tbsp Fresh or Dried Rosemary – (protects skin from free radical damage)

Base Ingredients:

½ cup Rosehip Seed Oil or Jojoba Oil – deeply hydrating and collagen-boosting

1 tbsp Beeswax (or Candelilla Wax for a vegan option) – thickens the Salve

5–10 drops of Frankincense Essential Oil – enhances skin regeneration

5–10 drops Lavender Essential Oil – calms and nourishes skin

Instructions:

Step 1: *Grind the Herbs in the Mortar & Pestle*

Add dried herbs to the mortar.

Using the pestle, grind them into a fine powder or paste.

This activates their skin-rejuvenating properties.

Step 2: *Infuse the Herbs into the Oil*

Transfer the ground herbs to a heat-safe bowl or small pot.

Pour rosehip seed oil or jojoba oil over the herbs until fully submerged.

Heat on low using a double boiler for 2–3 hours.

Stir occasionally.

Step 3: *Strain the Oil and prepare the Salve*

Strain using cheesecloth or a fine mesh strainer.

Melt beeswax in a small pot on low heat.

Stir in the infused oil and essential oils.

Pour into small tins or jars.

Let cool until solid.

How to Use: Apply daily to the face, neck, and hands for anti-aging benefits.

Creating your salves and balms at home is rewarding, allowing you to tailor formulations to your specific needs. Begin by making herbal-infused oils, a foundation for many skin care products. Steep dried herbs like calendula or chamomile in a carrier oil such as jojoba or almond for several weeks, allowing the beneficial compounds to infuse. This oil can be used as a nourishing moisturizer, offering the skin a dose of vitamins and antioxidants. For a facial steam, combine rosemary, lavender, and rose petals in a bowl of hot water. Lean over with a towel draped over your head to capture the steam, letting it open pores and detoxify the skin naturally. These steams are an invigorating way to refresh and prepare the skin for further treatments.

Face masks offer another avenue for rejuvenation. Blend powdered herbs like green tea or yarrow with honey or yogurt to create a revitalizing mask. Green tea, rich in antioxidants, fights free radicals and supports youthful skin, while yarrow enhances circulation and tones. Honey adds moisture and antibacterial properties, leaving the skin soft and radiant. For toners and hydrosols, use witch hazel or rose water. Witch hazel acts as a natural astringent, tightening pores and soothing irritation. Rose water hydrates and tones, reducing signs of aging with its antioxidant-rich petals. These toners provide a refreshing finish to your skincare routine, balancing the skin and preparing it for hydration.

Infused Dry Skin Repair Elixir Balm

This protective balm heals dry, damaged, or irritated skin.

Ingredients:

½ cup Shea butter – (deeply nourishing, helps skin elasticity)

¼ cup Calendula-infused oil – (speeds up wound healing)

¼ cup Rosehip-infused oil – (reduces scars and fine lines)

2 tbsp Beeswax or candelilla wax for a vegan version – (locks in moisture)

10 drops Lavender essential oil – (calms irritation and promotes healing)

10 drops Carrot seed essential oil – (boosts skin regeneration)

Instructions:

Melt shea butter and beeswax in a double boiler.

Remove from the heat and stir in the infused oils.

Add essential oils and mix well.

Pour into tins or jars and let cool.

Apply morning and night where needed.

Healing salves crafted with aloe, comfrey, or calendula offer a soothing balm for irritated or dry skin. Comfrey is particularly notable for containing allantoin, a compound that promotes cell regeneration and healing. This makes comfrey salves excellent for minor cuts and abrasions. Rosemary, with its antibacterial protection, stimulates circulation and reduces puffiness, making it a perfect addition to acne treatments; for those seeking to nourish their hair, herbal hair care rinses and oils can be made with infusions of nettle, known for its rich mineral content. These treatments fortify hair strength and vitality, providing a natural shine and resilience.

Proper application of these homemade remedies enhances their effectiveness. Massage infused oils gently into the skin, allowing them to absorb fully, and apply salves to affected areas using clean hands or a spatula. Choose the proper containers for storage, such as dark glass jars that protect contents from light and air exposure. Store these creations in cool, dark places to preserve their potency and extend shelf life. By crafting your skincare products, you harness the power of nature, offering your skin the purest form of care.

Making Salves and Balms for Skin Health

Creating salves and balms begins with understanding their foundational elements: oil infusion and natural thickening agents. At the heart of these soothing concoctions are infused oils, where herbs like calendula are steeped to extract their skin-soothing properties. This process involves immersing dried herbs in a carrier oil, such as olive or almond, allowing the oil to absorb the plant's healing compounds. Beeswax is a natural thickening agent, giving your salves and balms their solid form. Its gentle, waxy texture provides structure and adds a protective barrier to the skin, locking in moisture and enhancing the balm's effectiveness.

Mango Intense Hydration Moisturizing Salve

Deep hydration for skin repair.

Ingredients: *(Makes about 4 oz):*

Butters & Oils:

2 tbsp Shea Butter – deeply moisturizing, rich in vitamins A & E

2 tbsp Mango Butter – softens and smooths dry, rough skin

2 tbsp Jojoba Oil – mimics skin's natural sebum, helps regulate moisture

2 tbsp Rosehip Seed Oil – regenerates skin cells, evens skin tone

1 tbsp Avocado Oil – ultra-rich in fatty acids for deep repair

Waxes & Thickeners:

1 tbsp Beeswax (or Candelilla Wax for vegan option) – locks in moisture and adds a protective barrier

Optional Skin-Boosting Additions:

5 drops Lavender Essential Oil – calming and soothing

5 drops Frankincense Essential Oil – promotes skin regeneration

1 capsule Vitamin E Oil (optional) – antioxidant, extends shelf life

Instructions:

In a double boiler or heat-safe glass bowl over simmering water, melt: Shea butter, mango butter, jojoba oil, rosehip oil, avocado oil, and beeswax, stirring gently until fully liquid.

Remove from heat. Let cool slightly (until it is warm but not hot to the touch).

Stir in essential oils and vitamin E oil.

Whip with a hand mixer for 1–2 minutes or more for a fluffier Body Butter Texture.

Pour into sterilized glass jars or tins. Let cool and solidify fully before sealing.

How to Use:

Apply a small amount and warm it by rubbing it.

Massage into damp skin (after a shower is ideal!) for best absorption.

Use nightly on hands, feet, face, or anywhere prone to dryness.

Benefits:

✔ *Ultra-rich and non-greasy (with the right balance of wax to oils)*

✔ *Soothes eczema, dry patches, and flaking skin*

✔ *Forms a barrier to lock in moisture without clogging pores*

✔ *Naturally antimicrobial and anti-inflammatory*

Apply to dry skin as needed for long-lasting hydration and glow. Store in a cool place.

Oil infusion can be achieved through various methods, each offering its benefits. A slow infusion, using the gentle warmth of sunlight, is a time-honored technique that allows for a gradual extraction of the plant's essence. To do this, place your herbs and oil in a clear jar, seal it tightly, and leave it in a sunny spot for several weeks, shaking occasionally. This method, while requiring patience, respects the delicate nature of the herbs, ensuring a gentle and thorough infusion. Alternatively, a quicker method involves gently heating the oil and herbs in a double boiler, allowing for a faster extraction while maintaining the integrity of the plant compounds.

Formulating your salves and balms involves combining these infused oils with beeswax. Begin by melting the wax over a double boiler, creating a smooth, liquid base for your balm. Gradually add the infused oil, stirring gently to blend the two. Testing the consistency is key to achieving the perfect texture; a simple spoon-cooling method can help. Dip a spoon into the mixture and allow it to cool, then test its texture. If it's too soft, add more wax; if it's too firm, incorporate additional oil. This balance ensures that your salve or balm spreads easily and provides the desired level of protection and nourishment.

Egyptian-Inspired Beard Balm

Natural Nourishment & Grooming for Men

Ingredients:

1 tbsp beeswax (natural styling hold)

1 tbsp shea butter (deep hydration)

1 tbsp jojoba oil (strengthens and conditions)

1 tsp argan oil (promotes beard health and softness)

5 drops of cedarwood essential oil (woodsy aroma and promotes growth)

3 drops sandalwood essential oil (soothing and aromatic)

Instructions:

Melt beeswax and shea butter gently over low heat.

Remove from heat, stir in jojoba and argan oils.

Add essential oils and blend well.

Allow mixture to cool slightly, pour into a container, and let solidify.

Benefits:

- ✔ *Conditions & softens beard*
- ✔ *Tames and shapes hair*
- ✔ *Supports healthy beard growth*
- ✔ *It provides a pleasant, masculine fragrance*
- ✔ *Embrace timeless grooming inspired by Egyptian tradition.*

~

Specialized recipes cater to common ailments, showcasing the versatility of these skin remedies. For sore muscles, an anti-inflammatory arnica salve can provide relief. Infuse arnica flowers in oil, blend with beeswax, and add a few drops of essential oil like peppermint for a cooling effect. This salve is perfect for massaging into aching muscles, offering comfort and reducing inflammation. Lavender balm, known for its calming properties, is ideal for irritated or sensitive skin. Infuse lavender buds in oil and incorporate this soothing blend with beeswax to create a balm that calms and hydrates. This balm can be used to soothe minor skin irritations, providing a gentle, restorative touch.

Crafting salves and balms is as much about the journey as the result. It involves a dance of patience and intuition, a connection to the plants you nurture, and the healing they offer. As you experiment with these formulations, you become attuned to their subtleties, adjusting and refining them to suit your unique needs. Through this practice, you create products that care for your skin and cultivate a deeper understanding of the relationship between nature and well-being. Each balm and salve becomes a testament to the power of plants, a reminder of the wisdom within the garden and ourselves.

Adapting Remedies for Children's Needs

Children present unique challenges and opportunities when it comes to herbal remedies. Their bodies are still developing, requiring special considerations to ensure safety and efficacy. The key lies in tailoring remedies to their specific needs and adjusting dosages to align with their age and size. This requires a delicate balance. Too little might be ineffective, while too much can be harmful. It's crucial to begin with mild preparations and gradually increase as needed, always with an eye on the child's response. This approach ensures safety and fosters trust, making them more receptive to herbal treatments in the future.

Kid-Friendly Immunity Elixir

Gentle, tasty, and effective—this elixir is safe for children over 2 and uses sweet, calming herbs to build resilience without overpowering flavors.

Ingredients:

1 tbsp Dried Elderberries – antiviral and tasty

1 tsp Dried Chamomile Flowers – calms the nervous system, mild immune support

1 tsp Dried Rosehips – high in vitamin C

½ tsp Ground Cinnamon – warming and antimicrobial

½ tsp Fresh Ginger (grated or mashed) – immune-boosting and helps digestion

1 tbsp Raw Honey (omit for children under 1) – sweetens and soothes

½ tbsp Fresh Lemon Juice – brightens the flavor and adds vitamin C

2 cups filtered water

Instructions:

Crush the elderberries, chamomile, rosehips, and ginger using a mortar and pestle.

Add the herbal mash to a small pot with water and cinnamon, then bring to a low simmer for 20–25 minutes.

Strain and cool the liquid.

Once warm (not hot), stir in honey and lemon juice.

Store in a glass jar in the fridge for 5–7 days.

Dosage:

Ages 2–6: 1 tsp daily

Ages 7–12: 1 tbsp daily

During illness: every 4 hours as needed

It tastes like spiced berry tea with honey — gentle and yummy!

Crafting remedies for children involves creativity and an understanding of their preferences. Chamomile and honey sleep syrup is a favorite, combining chamomile's soothing properties with honey's natural sweetness. This gentle syrup can ease children into sleep, calming restless minds and bodies. Herbal popsicles and lollipops offer another avenue for immune support and comfort. Treats infused with kid-friendly herbs like elderberry or echinacea provide taste and health benefits, making medicine a delightful experience. Herbal bath blends for relaxation can also be a part of their routine, transforming bath time into a calming ritual that prepares them for restful sleep.

Mild Nighttime Bath Soak Elixir for Kids

Safe for ages 2 and up, and perfect for bedtime routines or after an overstimulating day.

***Ingredients** (One Bath):*

½ cup Epsom salt – provides magnesium to relax muscles and ease tension

¼ cup Baking soda – softens skin and neutralizes bath water pH

2 tbsp Dried Chamomile flowers – calming, anti-inflammatory, and gentle on young skin

2 tbsp Dried Lavender buds – promotes relaxation and sleep

1 tbsp Oatmeal (optional) – soothes sensitive skin and adds softness to the bath

2-3 drops Lavender Essential Oil (optional, age 2+ and well diluted)

Instructions:

Mix all dry ingredients in a bowl or jar.

Add essential oil only if using, and stir well to distribute evenly.

Scoop into a muslin bag, cotton sock, or tea infuser (to avoid herbs floating in the water).

Drop the bag into a warm bath and let it steep while the tub fills.

Soak for 15–20 minutes, keeping water warm—not hot.

Tips for Use:

✔ *Best used 30–60 minutes before bedtime*

✔ *Encourage quiet time after the bath: dim lights, storybooks, soft music*

✔ *Follow with gentle lotion or massage oil for added calming benefits*

Mild Nighttime Massage Oil Elixir for Kids

After the bath, massage the feet and back with:

2 tbsp Sweet Almond Oil, Jojoba Oil, Olive Oil, or Coconut Oil

Store oil infused with Dried Chamomile flowers for an enhanced calming effect.

Mix well and warm slightly in the hands before use.

When using herbs with children, safety must always be the priority. Certain herbs, strong tinctures, and essential oils can be too potent for young systems and should be avoided. Consulting with a pediatrician or a qualified herbalist can guide which herbs are appropriate and safe for use. This ensures you are informed about any potential interactions with medications or conditions. Education and caution are your allies in this endeavor, allowing you to introduce herbal remedies with confidence and care.

Immunity Elixir Tea Hack

If you're short on time:

Place all dry herbs (elderberries, rosehips, chamomile) into a tea infuser or muslin bag.

Steep in hot water for 10–15 minutes, add honey and lemon.

Quick and easy on-the-spot immune tea!

Making herbal remedies appealing to children involves engaging their senses and imagination. Fun packaging and flavors can transform a simple remedy into something they look forward to. Brightly colored bottles or whimsical labels can make all the difference in their willingness to try a new treatment. Involving them in the preparation process can also cultivate interest and acceptance. Allow them to help measure ingredients or stir mixtures, turning the creation of remedies into a bonding activity. This hands-on approach demystifies the process and empowers them with a sense of ownership and curiosity.

Turn Elixirs Into Gummies

- ✔ *Mix ½ cup elixir with 2 tbsp grass-fed gelatin, let bloom, then heat gently until dissolved.*
- ✔ *Pour into silicone molds, chill until firm.*

Fun & effective for kids (and grown-ups, too!)

As you navigate the world of herbal remedies for children, remember that patience and adaptability are key. Each child is unique, and what works for one may not work for another. Observing their reactions and adjusting ensures that their needs are met effectively and safely. Through careful attention and creativity, you can introduce them to the wonders of herbal medicine, laying the foundation for a lifelong appreciation of natural healing.

Crafting these remedies enriches your family's health with nature's bounty. As you turn the page to the next chapter, you'll explore integrating apothecary practices into your daily life, enhancing your journey toward holistic wellness.

Chapter Six
Integrating Apothecary Practices into Daily Life

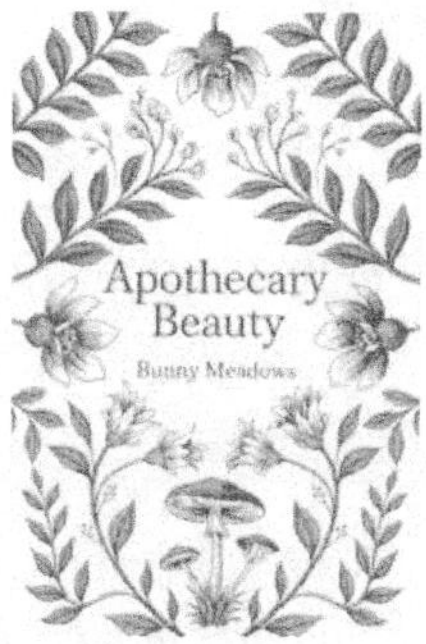

The first rays of sunlight touching the earth are a perfect setting to embrace the calming ritual of herbal wellness. This chapter invites you to create a routine that resonates with your rhythms and enhances your well-being. In a world where the pace of life can be overwhelming, establishing a consistent herbal routine becomes a beacon of tranquility and vitality. It is an opportunity to realign with nature, harnessing the power of herbs to elevate your energy levels, sharpen your mental clarity, and impart a youthful glow that radiates from within. By integrating herbs into your everyday practices, you nurture your body and cultivate a deeper connection to the natural world, creating a sanctuary of balance and harmony in your life.

Ayurvedic Intensive Hair Repair Salve

Ingredients:

¼ cup organic coconut oil

¼ cup organic shea butter

2 tbsp organic castor oil

1 tbsp organic Brahmi powder

1 tbsp organic Amla powder

1 tbsp organic Bhringraj powder

10 drops of lavender essential oil

5 drops of rosemary essential oil

5 drops of sandalwood essential oil

Directions:

Gently melt coconut oil and shea butter together over low heat.

Remove from heat, and stir in castor oil, Brahmi, Amla, and Bhringraj powders until thoroughly blended.

Allow the mixture to cool slightly, add essential oils, and stir thoroughly.

Transfer to a clean, sterilized glass container and let cool completely until solidified.

Benefits:

- ✔ *Deeply nourishes and strengthens hair follicles*
- ✔ *Supports hair growth and thickness*
- ✔ *Repairs damage, reduces split ends, and conditions dry hair*
- ✔ *Provides calming aromatherapy effects*

Use: Massage a small amount into scalp and hair lengths, and leave overnight or for at least one hour before shampooing.

Storage: Store in a cool, dry place away from direct sunlight

A consistent herbal routine offers myriad benefits, enhancing overall well-being through regular interaction with the healing properties of plants. By infusing your day with herbs, you can improve your energy levels and mood, fostering a sense of vitality that carries you through life's demands. The gentle support of adaptogens, such as ashwagandha and Rhodiola, helps manage stress, balancing your body's response to daily challenges and promoting a state of equilibrium. These herbs stabilize your mood, offering a calm assurance as you navigate the ebbs and flows of life. Enhanced mental clarity is another boon of a regular herbal practice. Cognitive-supportive herbs like ginkgo biloba and bacopa monnieri sharpen your focus and concentration, empowering you to approach tasks with renewed sharpness and efficiency. These herbs nourish your mind and contribute to a glowing, vibrant appearance, a testament to the inner balance achieved through mindful herbal integration.

Ginkgo & Bacopa Cognitive Clarity Elixir

A smooth daily tonic to energize your mind and sharpen your memory.

1 cup hot water

1 tsp dried ginkgo biloba leaves

½ tsp fresh grated ginger

Steep for 10 minutes and strain

Add ½ tsp bacopa powder (start small — it is potent and slightly bitter)

1 tsp raw honey or maple syrup

1 tsp lemon juice (vitamin C for antioxidant support)

Optional: splash of oat or coconut milk for smoothness

Optional: pinch of cinnamon or cardamom for flavor and circulation

Selecting the right herbs for your routine is a personal journey shaped by your unique health goals and needs. Begin by identifying areas where you seek support, whether stress management, digestive health, or skin radiance. Adaptogens provide a cornerstone for those looking to manage stress, while digestive aids like peppermint and ginger relieve gut health. For skin healing and radiance, consider incorporating herbs such as calendula and aloe vera, which are known for their nurturing properties. Hormonal balance can be supported with herbs like red clover and chasteberry, providing gentle yet effective support. For immune resilience, echinacea and elderberry are reliable allies, boosting your body's defenses against seasonal challenges. By tailoring your herbal selections to your specific needs, you create a personalized apothecary that aligns with your wellness journey, fostering a sense of empowerment and self-sufficiency.

Nettle & Red Raspberry Leaf Estrogen-Support Tea

Nettle is rich in iron and minerals, while raspberry leaf supports estrogen regulation.

1 cup hot water

1 tsp dried nettle leaves

1 tsp dried red raspberry leaf

1 tsp honey

Steep for 10 minutes, strain, and drink.

Creating a daily herbal schedule is an art that blends structure with intuition, guiding you to weave herbs seamlessly into your life. Start your day with an energizing tonic like ginger and lemon tea to awaken your senses and prepare your body for the day ahead. Midday can be an opportunity to incorporate herbs that support mental clarity, perhaps through a refreshing peppermint tea or a ginkgo biloba supplement. As the day winds down, embrace calming rituals that soothe your mind and body. An evening chamomile infusion or a lavender bath can prepare you for restful sleep, signaling your body that it is time to unwind. This rhythm of herbal integration creates a harmonious flow, enriching your daily routine with moments of mindful nourishment.

Yarrow Bath Bomb for Skin Healing & Relaxation

A fizzy, herb-infused bath bomb that soothes inflammation, supports skin repair and promotes full-body relaxation.

Ingredients:

1 cup baking soda (softens skin and balances pH)

½ cup citric acid (creates the fizz and exfoliates)

½ cup Epsom salt (relieves muscle tension and replenishes magnesium)

½ cup cornstarch (binds ingredients and softens water)

2 tablespoons dried yarrow flowers, finely ground (for skin healing and circulation)

2 tablespoons carrier oil (e.g., coconut, almond, or jojoba oil)

1 teaspoon witch hazel or alcohol-free hydrosol (for moisture)

10 drops lavender essential oil (calming & skin-soothing)

5 drops of tea tree or chamomile essential oil (optional for antimicrobial and healing support)

Bath bomb molds (or use silicone molds or muffin tins)

Instructions:

Mix baking soda, citric acid, Epsom salt, cornstarch, and ground yarrow in a large bowl.

In a separate small bowl, combine carrier oil and essential oils.

Slowly add the wet ingredients to the dry, mixing continuously (to prevent fizzing).

Lightly spritz the mix with witch hazel a little at a time until it feels like moist sand and holds its shape when pressed.

Pack the mixture into molds firmly. Let sit for 24 hours to dry and harden.

Store in an airtight container and use within 3 months.

To Use:

For full skin and body benefits, drop one bomb into a warm bath and soak for 20–30 minutes.

Benefits:

✔ *Soothes Irritated or Inflamed Skin – Yarrow calms and supports healing.*

✔ *Eases Muscle Tension – Epsom salt and essential oils promote relaxation.*

✔ *Cleanses & Softens Skin – Baking soda and oils gently cleanse and hydrate.*

✔ *Aromatherapeutic – Lavender and chamomile promote peace and emotional balance.*

~

Consistency is key to maintaining an effective herbal routine; a few strategies can help you stay on track. Set reminders on your phone or calendar to prompt you to take your herbal preparations, ensuring they become a regular part of your day. Placing herbal teas and tinctures in visible areas of your kitchen serves as a gentle nudge, reminding you to incorporate them into meals and snacks. By integrating these practices into your daily life, you foster a sense of ritual and reverence for the healing power of herbs, enhancing your connection to nature and yourself.

Interactive Element: Herbal Routine Journal

To further deepen your engagement with your herbal routine, consider maintaining a journal dedicated to your herbal practices. Record your daily herbal intake, noting any changes you observe in your well-being, mood, and energy levels. Reflect on how each herb resonates with you, and adjust as needed to better align with your evolving needs. This practice enhances your awareness of the benefits of herbs and empowers you to take an active role in your health and wellness journey.

Mindfulness and Herbalism: A Symbiotic Relationship

Imagine the serene ambiance of a quiet morning, where brewing a cup of herbal tea transforms into a mindful ritual. Mindfulness and herbalism intertwine, fostering a holistic approach to health that nurtures both body and spirit. Mindful tea ceremonies offer a moment to pause and connect deeply with the present. As you pour hot water over the leaves, watch the steam rise, carrying the essence of the herbs into the air. This simple act becomes a meditation, grounding you in the moment and opening your senses to the subtle qualities of the herbs. Each sip is savored, inviting a sense of calm and introspection. Similarly, meditative plant walks allow you to engage with nature at a slower pace. With each step, you become attuned to the textures and colors of the plants around you, absorbing the healing energy they offer. These practices enhance your connection to the natural world, cultivating inner peace and clarity.

Cordyceps Energy Tea Elixir

Enhances endurance, oxygen flow, and stamina—perfect as a morning or pre-workout drink.

1 cup brewed cordyceps tea

½ cup coconut water

1 tsp raw cacao powder

½ tsp maca powder

½ tsp honey

Pinch of cayenne (for circulation boost)

The role of intention in herbal preparation and use cannot be overstated. Setting a clear purpose before crafting or consuming remedies elevates the process, turning it into a focused and purposeful act. Before taking an herbal supplement, pause for a moment of mindful breathing. Inhale deeply, allowing your breath to fill your lungs, and exhale slowly, releasing tension and creating space for the herbs to work their magic. Visualization techniques during preparation further amplify this effect. As you blend your herbs, imagine the vibrant energy within each leaf and root, envisioning how it will support and nourish your body. This mindful approach imbues your remedies with a layer of personal intention, aligning them with your health goals and enhancing their effectiveness.

Pine Needle & Mint Detox Tea

Rich in vitamin C, this drink supports immunity and respiratory health.

1 cup hot water

1 tbsp fresh pine needles (chopped)

1 tsp dried peppermint

½ tsp lemon zest

1 tsp honey or maple syrup

Steep for 10 minutes, strain, and enjoy.

~

Certain herbs naturally lend themselves to mindfulness, offering support for mental clarity and emotional balance. Ginkgo biloba is renowned for boosting cognitive function, enhancing circulation, and reducing stress. Its leaves hold a wealth of compounds that promote mental acuity and resilience, helping you navigate life's demands with focus and grace. Lemon balm, with its gentle, lemony scent, uplifts the mood and eases anxiety, creating a sense of tranquility. It supports cognitive function, helping to clear the mental fog that often accompanies stress. Passionflower, known for its calming effects, quiets racing thoughts and promotes relaxation. It contains compounds that enhance GABA, a neurotransmitter that soothes the mind and fosters restful sleep. Valerian root, a potent natural sedative, eases tension headaches and alleviates muscle tightness. Its soothing properties make it a valuable ally in managing occasional anxiety and promoting deep, restorative sleep.

~

Ashwagandha & Cinnamon Adrenal Soothing Latte

A grounding and warming drink to regulate cortisol and reduce stress.

1 cup warm almond or oat milk

½ tsp ashwagandha powder

½ tsp cinnamon

1 tsp honey or maple syrup

Optional: ½ tsp coconut oil (for sustained energy)

The mental health benefits of integrating mindfulness with herbalism are profound. Together, they form a powerful synergy that reduces anxiety and depression. By grounding yourself in the present moment and supporting your body with herbs, you create a foundation for emotional well-being. These practices enhance focus and presence, allowing you to engage with your surroundings and relationships fully. The process of preparing and consuming herbs mindfully becomes a meditative experience, fostering a sense of calm and balance that permeates every aspect of your life. Through this integration, you cultivate a lifestyle attuned to nature's rhythms, promoting harmony within and without.

Nutrition Meets Nature: Holistic Wellness Framework

Envision your kitchen as a vibrant apothecary, where the harmony of herbalism and nutrition creates a foundation for optimal health. This synergy is a fusion of ancient wisdom and modern dietary practices, bringing a holistic approach to wellness. Herbs have long been revered for their ability to enhance nutrient absorption and complement meals in ways that elevate both flavor and function. Imagine starting your day with a breakfast that nourishes and prepares your digestive system to maximize nutrient uptake. By incorporating herbs into your meals, you tap into their potential to support your body's natural processes, profoundly impacting your overall health. Herbal teas, sipped throughout the day, offer another layer of support and work in tandem with your food to provide a gentle yet powerful enhancement to your dietary habits.

Parsley & Dandelion Power Bowl with Basil Pesto

A full-spectrum anti-inflammatory meal—fresh, earthy, zesty, and deeply nourishing

Base:

1 cup fresh flat-leaf parsley, chopped

1 cup young dandelion greens, chopped or torn

½ cup thinly sliced fennel

½ cup cucumber, diced

¼ cup red onion, thinly sliced

½ avocado, diced

½ cup cooked quinoa (or sprouted lentils or chickpeas for extra fiber/protein)

Toppings:

2 tbsp pumpkin seeds (zinc + crunch)

2 tbsp pomegranate seeds (optional for a pop of color and antioxidants)

1 scoop of basil pesto (see recipe above)

Optional: a few fermented veggies or a spoonful of sauerkraut

Basil Pesto Drizzle (from Chapter 1, Section 5):

2 cups fresh basil

¼ cup walnuts or hemp seeds

1 clove garlic

¼ cup olive oil

2 tbsp lemon juice

¼ tsp turmeric + pinch of black pepper

1 tbsp nutritional yeast (optional)

Sea salt to taste

Blend and drizzle generously.

Final Touch:

Squeeze of fresh lemon over everything
Cracked black pepper to finish
Optional: Top with a soft-boiled egg or grilled wild salmon for extra satiety

Pairing Tip:

Serve with a warm mug of rosemary and ginger tea for mental clarity and circulation support.

Dandelion, with its deep taproots, draws nutrients from the soil, making it a potent ally for detoxification. Its leaves can be added to salads, providing a bitter note that stimulates digestion and encourages the liver's natural cleansing processes. Dandelion leaves picked before the plant flowers will be sweeter. Cinnamon, a common household spice, goes beyond flavor enhancement. It plays a crucial role in blood sugar regulation, helping to maintain balanced energy levels throughout the day. Sprinkle it over oatmeal or blend it into smoothies for a sweet, spicy boost. Parsley, often relegated to the role of garnish, deserves a more prominent place in your diet. Its high vitamin C content supports tooth and gum health and can be chopped into salads or blended into pestos. These herbs, while simple, offer targeted support for various nutritional needs, demonstrating the profound impact of integrating herbalism into your daily meals.

Banana Nut Herbal Ice Cream

A creamy, naturally sweet ice cream with the grounding energy of bananas and the nourishing crunch of nuts—perfect for vitality and comfort.

Ingredients:

3 ripe bananas, sliced and frozen

½ cup full-fat coconut milk (or almond milk for a lighter texture)

¼ cup walnuts or pecans, roughly chopped (for omega-3s and crunch)

2 tablespoons nut butter (almond or peanut for richness)

1–2 tablespoons maple syrup or raw honey (optional, depending on sweetness)

½ teaspoon vanilla extract (for warmth and depth)

½ teaspoon cinnamon (for blood sugar balance and flavor)

Pinch of sea salt (to enhance flavor)

Optional Herbal Add-Ins:

1 teaspoon maca powder (for energy and hormone balance)

1 teaspoon ashwagandha (for a calming adaptogenic twist)

Instructions:

Combine frozen banana slices, coconut milk, nut butter, vanilla, cinnamon, and salt in a blender or food processor.

Blend until smooth and creamy.

Stir in chopped nuts and any optional herbs.

Transfer to a freezer-safe container and freeze for 1–2 hours for a scoopable texture, or enjoy immediately as soft-serve!

Let it sit at room temperature for 5–10 minutes before scooping if it is frozen solid.

Benefits:

✔ *Potassium & Fiber Rich – Bananas support heart and digestive health.*

✔ *Protein & Healthy Fats – Nuts provide lasting energy and nourishment.*

✔ *Adaptogenic Options – Maca and ashwagandha elevate this dessert into a wellness-enhancing treat.*

✔ *Refined Sugar-Free & Dairy-Free – Gentle on digestion and blood sugar.*

~

Consider the transformative potential of herbs as you explore recipes that seamlessly incorporate their benefits into everyday dishes. A herbal-infused salad dressing can elevate a simple salad to a healing meal. Blend olive oil with apple cider vinegar, add minced garlic, and whisk in fresh herbs like basil and oregano. This dressing enhances flavor and delivers anti-inflammatory benefits, particularly when paired with leafy greens. A turmeric-spiced quinoa salad becomes a culinary delight and a source of inflammation-fighting compounds. Cook the quinoa with turmeric, then toss it with roasted vegetables and a squeeze of lemon juice for a vibrant dish that supports joint health. Sage-infused chicken broth simmered becomes a nourishing tonic during cold months, supporting immune function and soothing the soul.

~

Warm Sweet Potato Healing Superfood Bowl

Comforting, cleansing, and nutrient-rich.

Earthy Base:

1 cup steamed sweet potato, cubed (deeply nourishing, rich in beta-carotene and grounding energy)

½ cup cooked quinoa (gentle on digestion, complete protein)

½ cup lightly sautéed dandelion greens or kale (bitter greens to support the liver and lymphatic flow)

½ cup steamed broccoli (supports detox, sulforaphane-rich)

The Healing Toppings:

½ avocado, sliced (soothing fats, brain and skin nourishment)

¼ cup roasted chickpeas or sprouted lentils (adds texture and gut-friendly fiber)

2 tbsp basil pesto (see Meadow Bunny pesto recipe—herbal, anti-inflammatory, vibrant)

1 tbsp tahini or olive oil drizzle (healthy fats to absorb fat-soluble vitamins)

1 tbsp pumpkin or hemp seeds (zinc, magnesium, mineral support)

Optional: a spoonful of fermented carrots or sauerkraut (gut flora support, tangy balance)

Healing Dust:

½ tsp turmeric + pinch of black pepper (synergistic anti-inflammatory magic)

A sprinkle of cumin, smoked paprika, or cinnamon (warming spice, supports digestion and circulation)

Optional: a touch of sea salt and fresh cracked pepper to balance the flavors

Finish:

A fresh lemon wedge (vitamin C + brightens the bowl)

Torn parsley, cilantro, or microgreens for vitality and color

Optional: sprinkle of nutritional yeast for B vitamins and umami

Pairing Suggestion:

Sip with a warm mug of ginger-nettle tea or a comforting ashwagandha and oat straw infusion to restore the nervous system and soothe the spirit.

~

In smoothies, herbs like mint and basil can add unexpected depth and freshness. Blend them with fruits and vegetables for a nutrient-rich drink that revitalizes the body. Herb garnishes, often overlooked, can transform a dish from ordinary to extraordinary. Parsley sprinkled over soups or mint leaves scattered in desserts adds visual appeal and contributes to your nutritional intake. Basil, with its aromatic leaves, forms the foundation of a nutrient-rich pesto. Combine it with pine nuts, garlic, and Parmesan for a versatile sauce that can be stirred into pasta or spread over toast. Rosemary, roasted with vegetables, enhances digestion and adds an earthy, fragrant note that ties the meal together.

Creating a balanced diet with herbal support requires thoughtful planning. Begin by considering your weekly meal prep and incorporating herbs into your menus. Pair herbs with seasonal produce to maximize their benefits and enjoy the freshest flavors. As you plan your meals, consider how each dish can contribute to your overall health goals. By weaving herbs into your dietary routine, you enrich your meals and embrace a lifestyle that honors nature's wisdom. This approach fosters a deeper connection to your food and the earth, nurturing both body and spirit as you embrace the holistic potential of nutrition and herbalism.

Using Herbal Teas for Daily Balance

As the world slowly awakens, a simple herbal tea can set the tone for the day ahead. The versatility of herbal teas lies in their ability to address various health aspects, offering benefits ranging from digestive support to stress reduction. For centuries, these infusions have been cherished for their gentle healing properties. A soothing peppermint tea we explored can ease digestive discomfort, relax the digestive tract muscles, and reduce bloating and gas. This same natural menthol in peppermint acts as a muscle relaxant, helping relieve tension headaches and migraines. This refreshing brew is a testament to the power of herbs, providing relief and comfort with each sip. For those seeking a calming end to the day, an evening blend of chamomile and valerian root offers a powerful remedy for stress relief and sleep support. These herbs work in harmony to calm the nervous system, promoting deep rest and relaxation.

Selecting the right herbal teas involves considering your specific health goals and time of day. Energizing blends, like ginger and lemongrass, are ideal for morning consumption. Ginger is a staple in traditional medicine, renowned for supporting digestion, boosting immunity, and enhancing overall well-being. Lemongrass adds a citrusy note, uplifting the senses and invigorating the spirit. Together, they create a vibrant tea that awakens the body and mind. As the day progresses, a rooibos chai with cinnamon and cloves offers a warming treat to boost energy and mood. Rooibos, naturally caffeine-free, is rich in antioxidants, while cinnamon and cloves provide a spicy warmth that comforts and revitalizes. For those moments leading into the evening, a passionflower and lavender blend can ease the transition from the day's busyness to a state of gentle calm.

Rooibos Radiance & Balance Tea

(A daily tonic for inner harmony + outer glow)

Ingredients:

1 tsp Rooibos tea (or teabag) – antioxidant + anti-inflammatory

1 tsp Nettle leaf – mineral-rich, supports hormones, and clears skin

½ tsp Shatavari powder (or 1 tsp dried root) – balances estrogen and supports feminine wellness

½ tsp Rose petals – cooling, heart-opening, and skin-calming

½ tsp Licorice root – adrenal support + skin-soothing (avoid if pregnant or with high blood pressure)

½ tsp Lemon balm – nervous system support and hormone-soothing

½ tsp fresh grated ginger – digestion, circulation, and immune boost

1 tsp honey or maple syrup

Splash of lemon juice (helps with absorption and brightness)

Optional: ½ tsp collagen powder or hibiscus for extra skin glow

Instructions:

Combine all herbs in a teapot or tea infuser.

Pour 1 cup hot water over them and steep for 10–15 minutes.

Strain, then stir in lemon juice and honey.

Add collagen or hibiscus if desired.

Sip slowly, ideally as a morning or early afternoon ritual.

Benefits:

✔ *Rooibos – reduces inflammation, rich in quercetin for skin & hormone balance*

✔ *Nettle – full of iron, silica, and skin-nourishing minerals; balances estrogen metabolism*

- ✔ *Shatavari – adaptogen for hormone harmony and hydration*
- ✔ *Rose – calms skin and heart, adds beauty inside and out*
- ✔ *Licorice root – supports adrenal recovery and clear, calm skin*
- ✔ *Lemon balm – reduces stress and helps regulate the menstrual cycle*
- ✔ *Ginger – supports immunity and circulation for healthy skin & scalp*

Brewing herbal teas is both an art and a science, where attention to detail enhances flavor and efficacy. The optimal steeping time and temperature can vary depending on the type of herb, with rooibos and herbal blends often requiring longer steeping times to release their flavors and beneficial compounds fully. It's important to use water that is appropriately heated to unlock the full potential of the herbs without burning them. For instance, black and herbal teas fare well with boiling water, while delicate herbs like chamomile or green tea may benefit from slightly cooler temperatures to preserve their subtle properties. Adjusting the steeping time can also help you tailor the strength of the tea to your preference, balancing the intensity of flavor and potency.

Transforming tea consumption into a mindful practice elevates the experience into a moment of daily meditation and relaxation. Create a calming tea-drinking space by selecting a cozy corner or a spot with a view of your garden, where you can savor the tranquility. Teapots or cups can enhance the sensory experience, adding a personal and aesthetic touch. Incorporate aromatherapy by diffusing essential oils that complement the tea's aroma, deepening the sensory connection between smell and taste. Light a candle or oil lamp. Set aside dedicated time for a daily tea meditation, allowing yourself to be fully present as you sip, appreciating the nuances of flavor and the warmth that spreads through your body. This ritual fosters a deeper connection to the herbs themselves and nurtures a sense of peace and mindfulness that can permeate your entire day.

Customizing Your Apothecary Experience

Your apothecary practice is as unique as you are, and personalizing it can transform your approach to wellness. Embrace the opportunity to create herbal blends that resonate with your specific needs and preferences. Whether you're seeking stress relief, immune support, or digestive harmony, crafting personalized herbal mixtures empowers you to address these goals directly. Start by selecting a few core herbs that align with your objectives. For instance, if relaxation is your aim, consider blending passion flowers, valerian, chamomile, lavender, and lemon balm. Experiment with proportions to find the perfect balance for your palate and purposes. This creative process enhances the effectiveness of your remedies and deepens your connection to the plants and their healing properties.

Calendula Petal & Coconut Cream Dessert

A delicate, floral-infused, dairy-free treat for beauty and digestion.

Ingredients:

1 can full-fat coconut milk

2 tablespoons dried calendula petals

2 tablespoons maple syrup or honey

½ teaspoon vanilla extract

1 tablespoon chia seeds (optional for texture and fiber)

Instructions:

Gently heat coconut milk over low heat, adding calendula petals.

Let simmer for 5 minutes, then remove from heat and strain petals.

Stir in maple syrup, vanilla, and chia seeds if using.

Chill in the fridge for 2-3 hours until thickened.

Serve with fresh berries or toasted coconut flakes.

Benefits:

✔ *Skin-nourishing*
✔ *Anti-inflammatory*
✔ *Digestion-friendly*

Creating unique herbal-infused oils is another avenue for personalization. These oils can serve as the base for salves, balms, or culinary delights. Begin by choosing a carrier oil, like olive or almond, that complements the herbs you wish to use. Gently heat the oil and add your selected herbs, allowing them to infuse over low heat for several hours. Once cooled, strain the mixture to remove plant material. The resulting oil will be rich with the essence of the herbs, offering a potent and versatile addition to your apothecary. Use these oils to enhance the flavor of dishes, nourish your skin, or as a massage oil to soothe tired muscles. The possibilities are vast and limited only by your imagination.

Glowing Skin Edible Oil Elixir

(Infused with herbs and skin-loving oils for beauty from within)

Base Oils (Organic and cold-pressed for internal use)

Choose 1–2:

All cold-pressed + organic for internal use:

Pumpkin seed oil – rich in zinc and vitamin E (supports hormones + skin elasticity)

Evening primrose oil – high in GLA (balances hormones, reduces acne + inflammation)

Hemp seed oil – omega-3s + anti-inflammatory, helps calm reactive skin

Olive oil (extra virgin) – antioxidant-rich carrier

Moringa oil – nourishing and skin-supportive

Infusion Botanicals (Dried, organic)

Use 1–2 tsp of each per 1 cup of oil:

Calendula petals – soothing, anti-inflammatory, promote skin healing

Rose petals – high in vitamin C, calming to the skin and heart

Gotu kola – supports collagen synthesis and circulation

Nettle – full of silica, iron, and skin-strengthening minerals

Chamomile – calms skin inflammation, eases digestive tension

Lemon balm – supports hormonal harmony and nervous system balance

How to Make It:

Place the chosen dried herbs in a clean, dry glass jar (fill about ⅓ of the jar).

Pour the base oil(s) over the herbs to completely cover.

Cap and shake gently.

Infuse for 3–4 weeks in a cool, dark place — shake gently daily.

(or do a quick warm infusion: heat in a double boiler on low for 2–3 hours)

Strain the oil through cheesecloth or fine mesh.

Store in a dark glass bottle away from heat and light.

How to Use (Internally):

Take 1 tsp daily by spoon or in warm tea

Add to smoothies, soup, porridge, or salad

Mix into warm oat milk with honey as a bedtime glow tonic

Optional Add-Ins:

A few drops of sea buckthorn oil for powerful skin renewal

Vitamin E oil for stability and added antioxidant support

A few drops of rosehip seed oil to use topically, too

Experimenting safely with herbs is crucial to a successful and satisfying apothecary practice. When introducing new herbs, start with small amounts to gauge how they affect your body. This cautious approach allows you to monitor your body's responses and make any necessary adjustments. Keeping a journal of effects and observations provides valuable insights into how different herbs work for you. Documenting your experiences helps refine your practices over time, ensuring that your herbal remedies remain effective and aligned with your evolving needs. This ongoing exploration fosters a sense of curiosity and discovery, encouraging you to deepen your understanding of each herb's unique properties and potential.

Self-awareness plays a pivotal role in customizing your apothecary experience. Understanding your health goals enhances your ability to select and use herbs effectively. Identify specific health markers to track, such as energy levels, mood changes, or skin conditions, and use these indicators to guide your herbal choices. Adjusting your herbal regimen based on seasonal changes can also be beneficial. For instance, in winter, you might focus on warming, immune-boosting herbs; in summer, cooling, hydrating herbs may take precedence. This dynamic approach ensures that your apothecary remains responsive to internal and external influences, supporting your well-being throughout the year.

Radiance Face Oil

A botanical infusion for glowing, calm, nourished skin

Base Oils (for all skin types):

Use light, non-comedogenic oils that absorb beautifully into the skin:

Jojoba oil – balances sebum, closest to the skin's natural oil

Argan oil, rich in vitamin E, protects and softens

Rosehip seed oil – brightens complexion, supports cell turnover

Meadowfoam seed oil – locks in moisture, extends shelf life

Optional: Sea buckthorn oil – powerful glow enhancer (use sparingly; it is vibrant orange!)

Infusion Botanicals (Same herbs as the edible oil):

Use dried herbs for infusing:

Calendula – healing + anti-inflammatory

Rose petals – toning, calming, add gentle fragrance

Gotu kola – collagen support + circulation

Chamomile – reduces redness and soothes sensitivity

Nettle or green tea – antioxidant and mineral-rich

How to Make It:

Fill a clean jar about ⅓ full with the dried herbs.

Pour the carrier oil blend over the herbs until fully submerged.

Cap and shake gently.

Infuse for 3–4 weeks in a cool, dark place (or low heat for 2–3 hours for a quicker batch).

Strain with cheesecloth or fine mesh.

Add optional actives:

Vitamin E oil (natural preservative)

A few drops of essential oil (see below)

Pour into dark glass dropper bottles.

Optional Essential Oils (5–10 drops per 1 oz):

Geranium – balances sebum, soft floral scent

Frankincense – skin toning, anti-aging

Carrot seed – regenerative, brightening

Lavender – calming for all skin types

Suggested Use: Massage 2–3 drops into clean skin after misting or serum. Use morning or evening.

As you engage with your apothecary practices, embrace the potential for growth and evolution. Try new herbs each season to expand your repertoire and discover new favorites. Attend workshops and join groups to connect with others who share your passion for herbalism. These interactions provide opportunities to learn from experienced practitioners, exchange ideas, and gain fresh perspectives. This continuous learning process enriches your understanding and keeps your practices vibrant and relevant. By remaining open to new experiences and information, you cultivate a flexible and adaptive approach that can evolve with your needs and interests.

In this chapter, we've explored how to integrate apothecary practices into daily life, emphasizing the importance of customization and self-awareness. This personalized approach enhances your health and deepens your connection to nature's wisdom. As you move forward, you'll discover that your apothecary is a living, breathing entity capable of adapting and growing with you. This sets the stage for the next chapter, where we'll delve into the art of ensuring safety and efficacy in your herbal practices, providing you with the tools to navigate the world of herbal medicine with confidence and ease.

Chapter Seven
Ensuring Safety and Efficacy

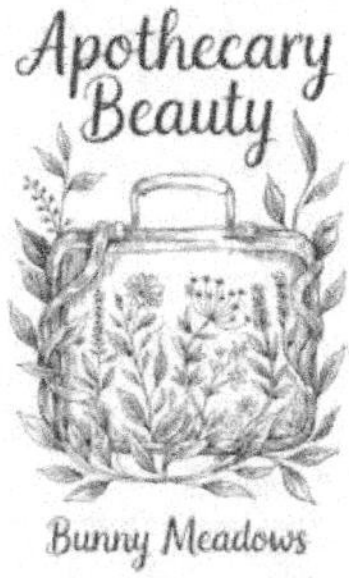

The sun begins to set over your garden, and the herbs you've carefully tended promise healing, a testament to the natural world's power to nurture and restore. With this potential comes the responsibility of ensuring that herbal remedies are used safely and effectively. Understanding dosage and potency is fundamental to this practice. It requires a blend of science and intuition as you learn to gauge the right amount of each herb for different purposes. This chapter explores these principles, offering you the tools to harness the full potential of your garden's bounty.

Hypericum Sleep & Stress Tincture

A potent extract for deep relaxation, nervous system support, and sleep aid.

Ingredients:

1 cup fresh hypericum flowers, chopped (or ½ cup dried)

1 ½ cups vodka or brandy (high-proof alcohol for extraction)

1 glass jar with lid

Instructions:

Fill a glass jar halfway with hypericum flowers.

Cover entirely with vodka or brandy.

Seal the jar and store it in a cool, dark place for 4–6 weeks, shaking occasionally.

Strain into a dark glass dropper bottle for storage.

Dosage: Take 10–15 drops with water or tea before bed for relaxation.

Benefits:

✔ *Supports sleep*
✔ *Eases anxiety*
✔ *Helps regulate mood naturally.*

Determining the appropriate dosage of herbs is both an art and a science. Several factors influence how much of a particular herb you should use. Age is a key consideration, as children and older people often require smaller doses than healthy adults. Weight also plays a role, with larger individuals typically needing higher amounts to achieve the desired effects. Health status is equally important. Those with chronic conditions or compromised immune systems might need to start with lower doses to avoid adverse reactions. By considering these factors, you can tailor your herbal treatments to suit individual needs, ensuring both safety and efficacy.

The form of the herb, whether fresh or dried, also affects dosage. Fresh herbs often contain more moisture, which can dilute their active compounds. You may need to use a larger quantity of fresh herbs compared to dried ones to achieve the same potency. Conversely, dried herbs are more concentrated, requiring careful measurement to avoid excessive doses. A general rule of thumb is to use three times the amount of fresh herbs as you would dry, but this can vary depending on the specific herb and its unique properties. Understanding these nuances allows you to optimize your preparations and maximize their therapeutic benefits.

Zinc-Rich Pumpkin Seed & Cacao Smoothie

Pumpkin seeds contain zinc, which is essential for maintaining hair health and balancing hormones, while cacao supports circulation and hair regeneration.

1 cup almond or oat milk

1 tbsp ground pumpkin seeds

1 tsp raw cacao powder

½ banana (for natural sweetness)

1 tsp honey

Ice cubes

Potency is another critical aspect of herbal medicine, influencing a remedy's effectiveness. The time of harvest can significantly impact potency. Many herbs are most potent at specific times of the year or during certain stages of their growth cycle. For example, leaves might offer the most benefits just before flowering. Similarly, roots are often richest in active compounds in the fall, when the plant's energy is concentrated below ground for winter survival. You can ensure that your herbs retain their maximum healing potential by timing your harvests carefully.

The methods you use to prepare your herbs also affect their potency. Techniques such as infusions, decoctions, and tinctures each extract different compounds, influencing the overall effectiveness of the remedy. Gentle methods like cold infusions may preserve more volatile oils, while decoctions can draw out mineral-rich compounds from tougher plant materials. Understanding these techniques allows you to choose the best method for each herb, aligning your preparation with the desired therapeutic outcome.

Lemon Balm & Valerian Root Herbal Ice Cream

A calming, creamy herbal dessert that soothes the nervous system, promotes relaxation and supports restful sleep.

Ingredients:

1½ cups full-fat coconut milk (or your preferred plant-based milk)

½ cup cashew cream or soaked cashews (for creaminess)

¼ cup raw honey or maple syrup (natural sweetener)

2 tablespoons dried lemon balm (nervine and mood-lifting)

½ tablespoon dried valerian root (supports sleep and eases tension)

1 teaspoon vanilla extract (for warmth and depth of flavor)

Pinch of sea salt (enhances flavors)

Optional: 1 teaspoon lemon zest (for brightness)

Instructions:

In a saucepan, combine coconut milk with lemon balm and valerian root.

Heat gently over low heat for 15–20 minutes, careful not to boil.

Strain out the herbs and allow the infused milk to cool.

Blend the infused milk with cashew cream, honey/maple syrup, vanilla, salt, and lemon zest until smooth.

Chill the mixture in the refrigerator for 1–2 hours.

Pour into an ice cream maker and churn according to the manufacturer's instructions.

No ice cream maker? Pour into a freezer-safe container and stir every 30 minutes until set.

Freeze until firm, then sit for 5–10 minutes before serving.

When adjusting dosages, it's wise to start with the minimum effective dose. This cautious approach reduces the risk of adverse effects and allows you to observe how your body responds. Gradual adjustments, increasing the dose incrementally, help you find the sweet spot where benefits are maximized without unintended consequences. This methodical approach ensures that you use herbs responsibly, respecting their power while harnessing their benefits.

A common misconception is that "more is better" when it comes to herbal remedies. This belief can lead to overdosing, which is particularly risky with potent herbs like St. John's Wort. This herb, often used for its antidepressant properties, can cause serious side effects if taken in excessive amounts, including photosensitivity and interactions with medications. By challenging this misconception, you embrace a more balanced approach emphasizing moderation and mindfulness in your herbal practice.

Visual Element: Herbal Dosage Chart

Consider creating a dosage chart for used herbs. Include columns for fresh and dried forms and notes on potency variations due to harvesting and preparation methods. This chart can serve as a handy reference, helping you make informed decisions about dosages and ensuring that your herbal remedies are safe and effective. By incorporating this tool into your apothecary, you deepen your understanding of dosage principles, enhancing your confidence in using herbs to support health and well-being.

Avoiding Harmful Interactions Between Herbs

Plants hold promise and potential, but an intricate dance exists between them. While herbs offer myriad benefits, they can also interact with one another and with medications, sometimes in ways that might not be immediately apparent. This is especially true for herbs that can either amplify or weaken the effects of others. For example, combining ginseng with certain blood pressure medications can enhance or reduce their effectiveness, leading to unexpected results. Blood-thinning medications, in particular, require careful consideration. Garlic, ginger, and ginkgo, while beneficial, can increase the risk of bleeding when taken alongside anticoagulants like warfarin. Understanding these interactions is crucial for safety and efficacy in herbal practice.

Heirloom Pepper Elixir for Metabolism & Immunity

A vibrant, antioxidant-rich elixir crafted with heirloom peppers to support metabolism, circulation, and immune function.

Ingredients:

2 heirloom sweet peppers (red, orange, or yellow for vitamin C and antioxidants)

½ red chili pepper (optional, for metabolism-boosting capsaicin)

½ cup carrot juice (for added beta-carotene and skin nourishment)

1 tablespoon apple cider vinegar (for digestion and detox support)

½ teaspoon turmeric powder (for anti-inflammatory benefits)

1 teaspoon raw honey (optional, for natural sweetness and immune boost)

¼ teaspoon black pepper (enhances turmeric absorption)

½ teaspoon fresh lemon juice (for vitamin C and alkalizing effects)

1 cup coconut water or filtered water (for hydration and electrolyte balance)

Instructions:

Wash and chop the heirloom peppers, removing seeds if preferred.

Juice all ingredients using a juicer. (If using a blender, blend all ingredients and strain through a nut milk bag or fine mesh strainer.)

Stir in turmeric, black pepper, and honey (if using).

Serve chilled for a refreshing, metabolism-boosting tonic.

Benefits:

✔ *Rich in Vitamin C & Antioxidants – Heirloom peppers support immune function and skin health.*

✔ *Boosts Metabolism & Circulation – Capsaicin in chili peppers enhances fat-burning and cardiovascular health.*

✔ *Supports Digestion & Detoxification – Apple cider vinegar and lemon aid in gut health.*

✔ *Anti-Inflammatory & Hydrating – Turmeric, coconut water, and peppers reduce inflammation and promote hydration.*

To navigate these complexities, adopting strategies to minimize risks becomes vital. A detailed log of your herbs and medications can be a valuable reference tool. Note the specific herbs, their doses, and any medications you take. This record helps identify potential interactions and provides a clear picture of your regimen, making it easier to share with healthcare providers or herbalists. Consulting with holistic professionals bridges the gap between herbal and conventional medicine. Their insights can highlight possible interactions and suggest modifications to your herbal routine, ensuring you benefit from your garden's bounty without unintended consequences.

Timing plays a pivotal role in managing interactions. The sequence in which you consume herbs and medications can influence their effects. Some interactions might be avoided by staggering intake. For instance, taking a particular herb a few hours apart from a medication can reduce the risk of interactions, allowing each to work independently without interference. This approach requires a thoughtful understanding of each herb's properties and interactions with other substances. By being mindful of timing, you can optimize the benefits of your herbal remedies while reducing potential risks.

Sage Hormone-Balancing Meat & Vegetable Rub

A nutrient-rich, aromatic rub designed to support hormonal balance, enhance metabolism, and add deep herbal flavor to meats and roasted vegetables.

Ingredients:

1 tablespoon dried sage (supports estrogen balance and digestion)
1 teaspoon rosemary (aids adrenal function and circulation)
1 teaspoon thyme (supports immune and hormone health)
½ teaspoon ground turmeric (anti-inflammatory and blood sugar balancing)
½ teaspoon black pepper (enhances nutrient absorption)
½ teaspoon cumin (aids digestion and supports hormone regulation)
½ teaspoon paprika (boosts circulation and metabolism)
½ teaspoon sea salt (mineral balance and adrenal support)
1 teaspoon garlic powder (supports detoxification and hormone health)
½ teaspoon onion powder (rich in sulfur compounds for liver detox)
1 teaspoon olive oil or avocado oil (optional for a wet rub)

Instructions:

Mix all dried ingredients in a small bowl or spice jar.
If making a wet rub, blend with olive oil or avocado oil.
Massage onto chicken, beef, lamb, or vegetables before roasting or grilling.
Let marinate for at least 30 minutes for a deeper flavor and benefits.

Benefits:

✔ *Sage & Rosemary – Support hormone balance, cognitive function, and adrenal health.*

✔ *Turmeric & Black Pepper – Aid inflammation reduction and blood sugar regulation.*

✔ *Thyme & Garlic – Assist in liver detox, crucial for hormonal balance.*

✔ *Paprika & Cumin – Boost circulation and metabolism for energy regulation.*

Making informed decisions is the cornerstone of safe herbal use. Educating yourself about potential interactions empowers you to take charge of your herbal practices. Relying on reputable sources for information is essential. Online resources, academic journals, and trusted herbal compendiums provide insights into known interactions and offer guidance on safe usage. These resources act as a safety net, backing your decisions with evidence and expert advice. Researching and understanding interactions cultivates a deeper connection to your herbal practice, enhancing your confidence and competence.

The landscape of herbal interactions is vast, but you can navigate it successfully with awareness and vigilance. Each herb in your garden carries its own set of characteristics and potential interactions. By respecting these intricacies, you honor the power and complexity of nature. As you continue to explore the therapeutic potential of your herbs, remember that safety is paramount. Balancing curiosity with caution ensures that your herbal practice remains a source of healing and well-being, enriching your life with each carefully chosen remedy.

Recognizing Signs of Adverse Reactions

Picture yourself enjoying the soothing scent of lavender from your garden, only to notice a sudden itchiness. This could be an allergic reaction, a typical adverse response to certain herbs. Recognizing these signs is vital for anyone engaging with herbal remedies. Allergic reactions can manifest as skin rashes, hives, or itching, often shortly after exposure. Gastrointestinal distress, such as nausea or diarrhea, might also occur, signaling that an herb does not agree with your system. These reactions are your body's way of communicating discomfort, urging you to pay attention and take action.

~

Libido-Enhancing Essential Oil Blend

Stimulating and hormone-regulating aromatherapy blend for libido and reproductive energy.

Ingredients:

5 drops Ylang Ylang essential oil – enhances libido and reproductive energy

5 drops Clary Sage essential oil – supports estrogen balance

5 drops Rose essential oil – increases sensuality and circulation

1 tbsp Jojoba oil (carrier oil)

Instructions:

Mix essential oils in a small glass bottle.

Apply a few drops to the wrists, neck, or abdomen daily.

Inhale deeply for hormone and mood balance.

~

Differentiating between adverse reactions and detox symptoms can be challenging, but it's crucial for your well-being. Detoxification symptoms, often mistaken for negative reactions, are typically temporary and mild, like a slight headache or fatigue. These occur as your body expels toxins and adjusts to the new regimen. Adverse effects, on the other hand, are persistent and may worsen over time, such as ongoing nausea or persistent skin irritation. Understanding this distinction helps you respond appropriately, ensuring your herbal practice remains safe and beneficial. Awareness and mindfulness are your allies in navigating these experiences.

When faced with an adverse reaction, the first step is to discontinue the herb immediately. Listen to your body and act swiftly to prevent further discomfort. If the symptoms persist or escalate, seeking medical advice becomes imperative. A healthcare professional can help determine the cause and provide guidance on alleviating the symptoms. They can also identify any underlying issues that might have contributed to the reaction. This proactive approach ensures your safety and allows you to continue exploring herbal remedies with confidence and knowledge.

Endocrine Rejuvenation Bath Soak

A soothing bath soak to relax the endocrine system and reduce stress.

Ingredients:

1 cup Epsom salt – provides magnesium for adrenal function
½ cup Dried lavender – calms the nervous system
½ cup Dried chamomile – reduces cortisol and promotes relaxation
10 drops Clary Sage essential oil – supports hormonal balance

Instructions:

Mix all ingredients in a bowl.
Add to warm bathwater and soak for 20–30 minutes.
Use 1–2 times a week for stress and hormonal balance.

Monitoring and documentation are invaluable tools in managing your herbal use. Keeping a reaction journal allows you to track your experiences with different herbs, noting any adverse effects or unusual responses. Documenting the time, dosage, and specific symptoms helps identify patterns and pinpoint potential triggers. This record not only aids in personal understanding but also serves as an informative resource when consulting healthcare providers. Maintaining a thorough log empowers you with information that enhances your herbal practice, ensuring it aligns with your unique health needs.

Interactive Element: Reaction Journal Template

Consider creating a simple reaction journal template to help you document your herbal experiences. Include sections for the herb name, dosage, method of use, and any symptoms observed. Note the duration and intensity of each reaction and any other factors that might have influenced the outcome, such as diet or stress levels. This tool can guide you in making informed decisions about which herbs best suit your body, fostering a more personalized and effective approach to herbal medicine. Through careful observation and documentation, you gain deeper insights into the interplay between your body and the herbs you cultivate, paving the way for a more harmonious relationship with nature's gifts.

Safe Practices for Families and Pets

In the tranquil setting of your home garden, herbs offer a path to wellness for all ages, but special care is needed when sharing nature's gifts with children and older people. Their bodies process herbs differently, calling for careful adjustments to dosage and selection. For children, herbs like chamomile are gentle and soothing, yet even these require reduced doses to prevent overwhelming young systems. Older family members may benefit from herbs like ginger for digestion, but their slower metabolism necessitates cautious dosing. Some herbs, like peppermint, are invigorating but can be too stimulating for children and seniors. Avoiding potent herbs such as ginseng for these age groups is often wise, as their effects can be too strong. By tailoring herbal use to age, you ensure every family member can safely enjoy your garden's benefits.

Pets, too, can reap the rewards of herbal gardens when we consider their unique needs. Cats and dogs are particularly sensitive to certain plants, so choosing pet-safe herbs is crucial. Basil, parsley, and dill are non-toxic and can enhance your garden while offering pet health benefits, aiding digestion, and even repelling pests. Cats often enjoy the scent of mint or catnip, while dogs can benefit from chamomile, which soothes anxiety. But caution is necessary, as some herbs, like garlic and onions, are toxic to pets. Birds and rabbits also require special consideration; plants like lilies harm birds, while rabbits can be sensitive to herbs like yew. By focusing on safe, beneficial plants, you create a garden that supports the well-being of every creature in your care [Source 4].

Holistic Dog Biscuits (Base Recipe)

Herbal and nutrient-packed dog treats made with whole foods and love.

Base Ingredients (safe & nourishing):

2 cups oat flour (or whole wheat flour if not grain-sensitive)

½ cup pumpkin puree (digestion support and natural sweetness)

¼ cup unsweetened applesauce or mashed banana

1 egg

1 tbsp coconut oil or olive oil

1–2 tbsp herbal add-ins (see below)

Optional: 1 tsp flaxseed, turmeric, or ground chia for extra omega-3s and joint support

Herbal Options (Pick 1–2 depending on the benefit you want):

Calming:

Chamomile – anti-anxiety + digestion support

Lemon balm – soothes nerves, gentle on the tummy

Valerian root (tiny pinch) – natural sedative for anxious pups

Joint Support:

Turmeric – anti-inflammatory

Nettle – mineral-rich, helps reduce stiffness

Ginger – circulation + joint mobility

Skin & Coat:

Flaxseed – omega-3 fatty acids

Dandelion leaf – gentle detox + supports healthy skin

Oatmeal – soothing + fiber-rich

Immunity:

Astragalus (tiny pinch) – immune support

Rosehip powder – vitamin C-rich and anti-inflammatory

Parsley – breath freshening + immune boost

Instructions:

Preheat oven to 325°F (165°C).

Mix all ingredients into a dough. Add water if needed to make it pliable.

Roll out the dough and cut it into bone or heart shapes using cookie cutters.

Bake for 30–35 minutes until firm and golden.

Let cool completely before storing in an airtight jar.

~

Creating a safe herbal environment at home involves more than just choosing the right plants. Secure storage solutions are vital to prevent accidental ingestion by curious children or pets. Store dried herbs in high, locked cabinets and label them clearly to avoid confusion.

Consider raised beds or fencing in the garden to keep herbs out of reach of tiny hands and paws. A pet-friendly herbal garden can provide a safe space for exploration, using container gardens or vertical planting to protect delicate plants. Choosing locations that are less accessible to pets or children ensures that your garden remains a sanctuary for growth and healing, free of unintended risks.

Holistic Cat Treats (Base Recipe)

Soft-baked, herbal-infused bites for vibrant feline health

Base Ingredients (cat-safe & appealing):

½ cup cooked and mashed salmon, chicken, or tuna (or pumpkin for veggie version)

½ cup coconut flour or oat flour

1 egg

1 tbsp olive oil or salmon oil (for skin + coat)

1 tbsp catnip (for fun! optional)

1–2 tsp herbal boosters (see blends below)

Optional: 1 tbsp nutritional yeast (cats love the flavor + B vitamins)

Cat-Safe Herbal Add-ins by Benefit:

Calming:

Chamomile (tiny pinch)

Lemon balm – gentle, supports mood and digestion

Skin & Coat:

Dandelion leaf – detox + liver support

Flaxseed meal – omega-3s + hydration

Nettle – full of silica, iron, and minerals

Immunity + Vitality:

Catnip – fun + antioxidant-rich
Parsley – breath freshener + immune booster (small amounts only)
Rosehip powder – vitamin C-rich and anti-inflammatory

Urinary Support:

Cranberry powder (tiny pinch) – supports urinary tract health
Marshmallow root – soothes the urinary tract and digestion

Instructions:

Preheat oven to 325°F (165°C).

Mix ingredients into a soft dough. If it is too dry, add a splash of water or broth.

Roll into small balls or press into tiny cookie molds.

Bake for 10–15 minutes, until just set but soft.

Cool completely and store in the fridge for 5–7 days.

Education plays a pivotal role in maintaining safety within your herbal practices. Involving family members in the process fosters understanding and respect for the plants and their uses. Teaching children about safe plant handling is a valuable lesson in responsibility and care. Show them how to identify herbs, explaining which ones are safe to touch and which are not. Include them in simple preparation tasks, such as washing or arranging herbs, to build familiarity and interest. This involvement teaches safety and instills a sense of connection to the natural world and its cycles.

A family approach to herbalism also means sharing the joys and responsibilities of gardening and preparation. Encourage family members to participate in planting and tending to the garden, each contributing to its care. This collaborative effort strengthens family bonds and fosters a shared appreciation for the natural world. As you work together, you create a living classroom where every member learns the value of nature's gifts, cultivating a culture of safety and mindfulness. In this way, your herbal garden becomes a haven of health and harmony, benefiting all who dwell within its embrace.

Myth-Busting Common Herbal Misconceptions

The gentle rustle of leaves whispers ancient secrets; it's easy to fall under the spell of nature's allure. The term "natural" often evokes images of purity and safety, yet this assumption can be misleading when it comes to herbal remedies. A prevalent misconception is that if something is natural, it must be safe. This belief overlooks the fact that many potent substances in nature can be harmful if misused. Plants like belladonna and foxglove contain compounds that are toxic in large amounts despite their historical use in medicine. Just because an herb grows in your backyard doesn't guarantee it's safe for consumption without proper knowledge and preparation.

The misunderstanding extends to the idea of herbal "cures." While herbs have been used for centuries to support health, they are not magic bullets that can cure every ailment. They work best as part of a holistic approach to wellness, complementing lifestyle changes and, when necessary, conventional treatments. It's vital to recognize that herbs can alleviate symptoms and support the body's natural healing processes. However, they are not a substitute for professional medical advice when dealing with severe health conditions. You can use herbs more effectively and responsibly by understanding the limits of what herbs can achieve.

Collagen & Moringa Hair Growth Latte

Collagen strengthens hair follicles, while moringa replenishes vitamins A, C, and E to encourage regrowth.

1 cup warm oat or almond milk

1 scoop collagen powder

1 tsp moringa powder

1 tsp honey or maple syrup

½ tsp cinnamon

Factual information and scientific research play a crucial role in dispelling these myths. Numerous studies document the benefits of herbs like turmeric and valerian, providing evidence for their anti-inflammatory and sedative properties. Historical data also support their use, tracing back to ancient civilizations that relied on plant-based medicine. Yet, even with this wealth of knowledge, it's vital to approach herbal remedies with a critical eye. Not every claim about herbs is backed by science; some are based on anecdotal evidence rather than rigorous study. You build a more reliable foundation for herbal practices by rooting your understanding in verified information.

The media and marketing industries often contribute to the spread of misconceptions about herbal remedies. Advertising campaigns can sometimes exaggerate the benefits of certain products, leading consumers to believe in miraculous outcomes. Terms like "detox," "superfood," and "natural cure" are frequently used to entice buyers, but these claims don't always hold up under scrutiny. It's essential to look beyond the marketing hype and investigate the evidence supporting these products. Misleading claims can lead to unrealistic expectations and disappointment, underscoring the need for discernment when navigating the world of herbal supplements.

Encouraging critical thinking and research is paramount in challenging these myths. Questioning the validity of claims and seeking out multiple sources of information can provide a more balanced perspective. Reputable herbal studies, academic journals, and credible health websites are invaluable resources. Consulting with knowledgeable herbalists or holistic healthcare professionals can offer insights grounded in experience and expertise. This approach enriches your understanding and empowers you to make informed decisions about your health.

Dandelion & Chicory Adrenal Coffee Alternative

A caffeine-free, liver-supportive blend that mimics the taste of coffee without adrenal stress.

1 cup brewed roasted dandelion root tea

½ tsp roasted chicory root

½ cup oat or almond milk

1 tsp maple syrup

¼ tsp cinnamon

As you continue your exploration of herbal medicine, remember that knowledge is your greatest ally. By equipping yourself with accurate information and remaining open to learning, you cultivate a safe and effective practice. This chapter has provided tools to navigate the complexities of herbal use, encouraging a thoughtful and informed approach. With this solid foundation, you are better prepared to embrace the healing potential of your garden, fostering a relationship with nature grounded in respect and understanding. As we move forward, the next chapter will guide you in exploring sustainability and environmental stewardship in your herbal practices, deepening your connection to the earth and its abundant gifts.

Chapter Eight
Sustainability and Environmental Stewardship

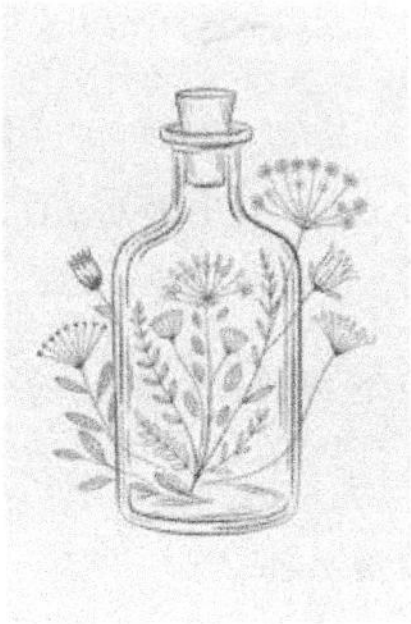

Picture your garden as a vibrant tapestry, where each plant and creature plays a crucial role in an intricate ecosystem. This image captures the heart of sustainability, a philosophy that extends beyond mere conservation to embrace holistic stewardship of our resources. As an adult gardener, you are uniquely positioned to nurture this balance, turning your apothecary practices into a force for positive environmental change. By adopting a zero-waste mindset, you can significantly reduce your ecological footprint, ensuring that your herbal endeavors leave a legacy of sustainability for future generations.

What Is Oil Pulling?

This is a beautiful, ancient Ayurvedic ritual for detoxifying the mouth and supporting gum and whole-body health. It is one of the most straightforward, most effective holistic oral care practices, and it is especially lovely when paired with thoughtful herbs or essential oils.

Oil pulling involves swishing oil in the mouth (like mouthwash) for 10–20 minutes to draw out toxins, reduce harmful bacteria, and nourish the gums.

Benefits of Oil Pulling

- ✔ *Strengthens gums and teeth*
- ✔ *Helps prevent cavities*
- ✔ *Reduces plaque and bacteria*
- ✔ *Freshens breath*
- ✔ *Supports detox through the mouth*
- ✔ *It may help whiten teeth naturally*

Zero-waste is more than a trend; it's a transformative approach to living that seeks to eliminate landfill waste by focusing on recycling, repairing, and composting. In a world where humans generate over 2.12 billion tons of waste annually, with 99% of purchased goods ending up discarded within six months, the impact of this philosophy is profound (Source 1). By embracing zero-waste in your herbalism, you actively contribute to a more sustainable future, ensuring that the resources we rely on are preserved for generations to come. This mindset challenges us to rethink our consumption habits, encouraging a more intentional approach to using and reusing materials.

How to Use Neem Twigs to Clean Teeth

1. Choose the Right Twig

Use a fresh, young twig from a neem tree (about 6–8 inches long and pencil-thick).

It should be green and flexible, not dried out or brittle.

2. Prep the Twig

Wash it thoroughly under running water.

Peel about 1 inch of bark off from one end.

3. Chew to Soften

Gently chew the peeled end until the fibers break apart and form a soft, brush-like fray (almost like natural bristles).

4. Brush Teeth

Use the frayed end to gently brush the teeth and gums, moving in small circular or vertical motions.

Spit out excess saliva.

5. Trim and Repeat

After brushing, cut off the used bristled end.

Reuse the stick the next day by chewing a fresh new end.

6. Spit, Rinse, Smile

Rinse mouth with water afterwards.

Enjoy the clean, bitter freshness—it may taste strong initially, but it is part of the cleansing action.

Benefits of Neem Twigs:

- ✔ *Antibacterial & antifungal: Helps fight plaque and gingivitis.*
- ✔ *Strengthens gums and soothes inflammation.*
- ✔ *Naturally, it whitens teeth and freshens breath.*
- ✔ *Biodegradable and sustainable alternative to plastic toothbrushes.*

One of the core tenets of zero-waste is reducing, reusing, and recycling. In the context of herbalism, this means minimizing waste during the preparation and storage of remedies. Utilizing reusable glass jars and containers is a simple yet effective strategy. These vessels preserve the potency of your herbal concoctions and reduce the need for disposable packaging. Composting plant waste and scraps further aligns with zero- waste principles, transforming what would be discarded into rich, nourishing soil that feeds future growth. By closing the loop in this way, you contribute to a cycle of renewal that sustains both your garden and the broader ecosystem.

Gum-Loving Herbal Toothpaste Recipe

Ingredients:

2 tbsp coconut oil – Antibacterial and soothing for inflamed gums

1 tbsp baking soda – Gently cleans and neutralizes acids

1 tbsp bentonite clay – Detoxifies and supports mineral balance

1 tsp myrrh powder – Powerful gum healer and antimicrobial

1 tsp clove powder – Eases gum pain, fights bacteria

½ tsp turmeric – Anti-inflammatory and brightening

5 drops tea tree essential oil – Potent antimicrobial (optional)

5–10 drops peppermint or spearmint essential oil – For freshness and breath

Optional: 1 tsp xylitol powder – A natural sweetener that also fights cavity-causing bacteria

Instructions:

In a non-metal bowl, mix coconut oil and baking soda until creamy.

Add bentonite clay, myrrh, clove, and turmeric, and stir well.

Add essential oils and xylitol if using. Mix thoroughly.

Store in a small glass jar with a lid.

Apply a small amount to the toothbrush using a clean spoon or spatula.

Gum Healing Benefits:

✔ *Myrrh: Speeds gum tissue healing and reduces bleeding.*

✔ *Clove: Numbs discomfort and kills bacteria.*

✔ *Turmeric: Soothes swollen or irritated gums.*

✔ *Coconut Oil: Fights bacteria and reduces plaque buildup.*

✔ *Tea Tree Oil: Targets bacteria deep in gum pockets.*

Mindful consumption is another pillar of the zero-waste philosophy, urging us to consider the origins and lifecycle of our products. As a herbalist, prioritizing local and bulk purchasing can drastically reduce packaging and transportation waste. Local herbs often require fewer resources to grow and transport, supporting sustainability and community resilience. Moreover, using every part of the plant—whether by incorporating stems into compost or using leaves in teas—ensures that nothing goes to waste. This intentional approach minimizes environmental impact and honors the plants, acknowledging their full potential.

Creativity plays a vital role in zero-waste practices, turning what might be considered refuse into valuable resources. Old cloth, for instance, can be repurposed into herbal sachets, providing a charming and sustainable way to store dried herbs. Empty bottles transform into decorative containers, adding aesthetic value while serving a practical purpose. Such practices embody the essence of upcycling, where materials are given new life and function. By viewing waste as an opportunity for innovation, you cultivate a mindset that values resourcefulness and sustainability, enhancing your apothecary practice with creativity and care.

Visual Element: Zero-Waste Apothecary Checklist

Consider creating a zero-waste apothecary checklist to guide your sustainable practices. List items such as reusable containers, composting methods, and upcycling ideas. As you implement these strategies, check off each item, noting the positive impact on your herbal practice and the environment. This visual tool tracks your progress and inspires continued commitment to sustainable living.

By weaving these zero-waste principles into your herbalism, you contribute to a more sustainable future. Your efforts, though seemingly small, ripple outward, influencing the broader ecosystem and inspiring others to follow suit. In doing so, you become a steward of the earth, nurturing its resources with intention and respect.

Biodiversity and Its Role in the Garden

Imagine your garden as a symphony of colors and textures, where each plant plays a distinct role in maintaining harmony. Biodiversity is the backbone of this balance, supporting a healthy ecosystem that thrives without the need for synthetic interventions. A diverse range of plants fosters natural pest control, as certain species repel unwanted visitors while others attract beneficial insects to keep pests in check. This natural balance reduces the need for harmful chemicals, ensuring your garden remains a haven for all creatures. Pollinators, essential for plant reproduction, are drawn to diverse gardens, where various blooms provide the nectar and pollen they need. By cultivating a rich tapestry of plant life, you create an environment where pollinators flourish, enhancing your garden's productivity. This interconnected web of life is crucial for the vitality of your apothecary, where each plant contributes to the ecosystem's overall health.

To increase biodiversity in your garden, start by planting a variety of herbs and companion plants. Each species brings unique benefits, from culinary uses to medicinal properties, enriching your apothecary with a spectrum of options. Companion planting involves strategically pairing plants that support each other's growth, creating a more resilient ecosystem. For example, planting basil alongside tomatoes enhances flavor and deters pests, while marigolds protect neighboring plants with their natural insect-repelling properties. Incorporating native species is another effective strategy, as these plants are well-adapted to local conditions and support indigenous wildlife. Native plants often require less maintenance and water, reducing the environmental impact of your garden. By embracing a wide range of plants, you foster a dynamic and resilient ecosystem that thrives in harmony with nature.

Holistic Collagen-Boosting Pudding Pops

A nourishing, creamy, frozen treat specifically crafted to naturally enhance collagen production, supporting skin elasticity, joint health, and overall wellness.

Ingredients (makes six popsicles):

1 ½ cups full-fat coconut milk (rich in healthy fats essential for collagen synthesis)

1 tablespoon chia seeds (omega-3s for skin hydration & elasticity)

1 tablespoon raw cacao powder (rich in antioxidants to protect collagen)

½ ripe avocado (provides vitamin E and healthy fats)

2 tablespoons grass-fed collagen powder (for additional collagen support)

1 tablespoon raw honey or maple syrup (skin-nourishing and naturally sweetening)

½ teaspoon vanilla extract (flavor and antioxidant-rich)

½ teaspoon rosehip powder or açai powder (optional for vitamin C and collagen production)

Pinch of sea salt (mineral support)

Instructions:

Combine coconut milk, chia seeds, cacao powder, avocado, collagen powder, honey/maple syrup, vanilla, rosehip/açai powder (if using), and sea salt.

Blend until smooth and creamy.

Due to chia seeds, allow the mixture to thicken slightly (5–10 minutes).

Pour into popsicle molds, insert sticks, and freeze for 4–6 hours or overnight.

To serve, run molds briefly under warm water and gently remove popsicles.

Benefits:

✔ *Boosts Natural Collagen Production – Vitamin C-rich rosehip/açai supports collagen synthesis.*

✔ *Skin Hydration & Elasticity – Chia, avocado, and coconut milk nourish skin cells.*

✔ *Rich in Antioxidants – Cacao and berries protect skin from free radicals.*

✔ *Supports Joint & Bone Health – Collagen powder supports extra connective tissue.*

Diverse ecosystems also enhance the medicinal qualities of herbs, as healthy soil and nutrient availability boost their potency. A biodiverse garden supports soil health by fostering a rich microbial community that aids nutrient cycling. This biological activity creates a fertile environment where plants can access the necessary nutrients, leading to higher concentrations of beneficial compounds. Furthermore, a diversity of plants creates synergistic effects, where certain species enhance the growth and potency of others. For instance, planting chamomile near mint can improve the latter's essential oil content, intensifying its therapeutic properties. This interplay between species enriches your apothecary, offering more potent remedies for beauty and wellness.

Regular observation and adaptation are key to maintaining biodiversity in your garden. Conducting biodiversity audits allows you to assess the variety of species and their interactions, providing insights into the health of your ecosystem. Adjusting your plant selection based on these observations, note which plants thrive together and which struggle. If certain species dominate, consider introducing new plants to balance the ecosystem, ensuring that no single species outcompetes the others. This adaptive approach encourages continuous learning and growth as you refine your practices to support a thriving, biodiverse garden. By embracing the principles of biodiversity, you not only enhance the health and productivity of your apothecary but also contribute to a more sustainable and resilient environment.

Sustainable Harvesting Techniques

Sustainable harvesting is deeply rooted in respect for nature's cycles, ensuring plants thrive and regenerate. By understanding and honoring these cycles, you protect plant populations and guarantee that your apothecary practice remains fruitful for years to come. Overharvesting poses a significant threat to plant communities, leading to depleted resources and the potential extinction of certain species. By taking only what you need, you preserve the integrity of these populations, allowing them to flourish. This practice is not just an ethical choice but a commitment to the environment that sustains us.

Cherry Pomegranate Dressing

(Sweet, tangy, and packed with skin-loving antioxidants)

Ingredients:

½ cup pomegranate juice (fresh or 100% pure)
¼ cup fresh or frozen cherries, pitted
2 tbsp apple cider vinegar (or balsamic for richness)
2 tbsp olive oil (or avocado oil for a silkier texture)
1 tbsp maple syrup (or raw honey)
1 tsp Dijon mustard (balances flavors and adds a little depth)
½ tsp fresh grated ginger (optional for a bit of zing and digestion support)
Pinch of sea salt and black pepper

Instructions:

Blend everything until smooth and creamy.

Taste and adjust—add more vinegar for tang and more honey for sweetness. Store in a glass jar in the fridge for up to 1 week.

How to Use It:

Salads: Toss with arugula, goat cheese, walnuts, and roasted beets.
Grain Bowls: Drizzle over quinoa, farro, or wild rice.
Glaze: Brush onto grilled tofu, salmon, or chicken.
Dip: Use as a dip for fresh veggies or spread on toast with avocado.

Respecting natural growth cycles involves recognizing when plants are at their peak and ready for harvesting. This not only maximizes the potency of the herbs you collect but also minimizes harm to the plant. For instance, just before flowering, harvesting leaves during their prime ensures you're gathering them at their most potent. Similarly, roots are best collected in the fall when the plant's energy is concentrated below ground. By aligning your harvesting practices with these natural rhythms, you support the plant's lifecycle, ensuring its continued vitality.

Ethical wildcrafting, the practice of harvesting plants from their natural habitats, demands a keen awareness of your surroundings and a commitment to sustainability. Start by identifying sustainable harvesting sites and areas where the plant population is robust and healthy. Avoid sensitive or endangered habitats, as these require protection and regeneration. When harvesting, always leave enough of the plant to regenerate and continue its lifecycle. A good rule of thumb is taking no more than one-third of a plant population, ensuring enough remains for regrowth and reproduction. This respectful approach conserves the plant's future and maintains the balance of the ecosystem.

Nourishing Skin Olive Tapenade

A luscious, skin-loving Mediterranean spread packed with antioxidants, healthy fats, and beautifying botanicals. This Olive Tapenade is a functional food that supports glowing skin, hydration, and cellular health. Thanks to omega-rich olives, skin-brightening lemon, and antioxidant-packed herbs, it's perfect as a spread, dip, or dressing base.

Ingredients:

1 cup mixed olives (Kalamata + Castelvetrano for a balance of flavors)
¼ cup extra virgin olive oil (cold-pressed, organic for maximum skin benefits)
2 tbsp capers (adds brightness and minerals)
1 tbsp lemon juice (rich in vitamin C for collagen support)
1 clove garlic (optional, for detoxifying and circulation-boosting properties)
1 tbsp hemp seeds (extra omega-3s for skin hydration!)
1 tbsp finely chopped walnuts or almonds (vitamin E boost for elasticity)
½ tsp fresh rosemary or thyme (anti-inflammatory and collagen-protecting)
½ tsp dulse flakes (or a pinch of sea salt) (natural iodine for skin and scalp health!)
Freshly ground black pepper (boosts absorption of antioxidants!)

Instructions:

Chop & blend: Pulse all ingredients together in a food processor until smooth or slightly chunky, depending on preference.
Adjust: Taste and add more lemon, olive oil, or herbs if needed.
Store: Keep in a sealed jar in the fridge for up to 1 week.

How to Enjoy It:

Salads – Toss with leafy greens, roasted veggies, or quinoa bowls.
Bread & Crackers – Spread over sourdough, pita, or seeded crackers.
Pasta or Noodles – Mix into warm pasta or spiral zucchini.
Avocado Toast Boost – Layer with avocado and hemp seeds for extra glow.
Protein Glaze – Spoon over grilled tofu or seafood.

Minimizing environmental impact during harvesting is crucial. Use non-invasive tools that cause the least disruption to the plant and its habitat. Sharp, clean pruners are ideal for cutting stems and leaves, as they reduce the risk of disease transmission and promote clean cuts that heal quickly. Target abundant populations where your harvesting will have the least impact. This strategy ensures that you're not taking from a dwindling resource but rather from a thriving one that can withstand the loss. By focusing on abundance, you help maintain ecological balance and protect vulnerable species.

Timing and technique are pivotal in sustainable harvesting. Early morning is often the best time to harvest herbs, as this is when they are most hydrated and their essential oils are concentrated. The coolness of the morning preserves these compounds, ensuring maximum potency. When harvesting, use sharp tools to minimize plant damage. Clean cuts encourage quick healing and reduce the risk of infection. This practice benefits the plant and enhances the quality of the herbs you collect, ensuring that they retain their therapeutic properties. Each plant has its own ideal harvesting time, so familiarize yourself with the specific needs of the species in your apothecary.

By integrating these sustainable harvesting techniques into your practice, you contribute to the health and resilience of the plant communities you rely on. This mindful approach ensures that your apothecary remains a source of healing and vitality for you and the environment. You nurture a harmonious relationship with nature through respect, knowledge, and care, where each harvest is a testament to your commitment to stewardship and sustainability.

The Impact of Climate on Herbal Growth

Climate serves as both a challenge and an ally, shaping the growth and potency of the plants you nurture in your herbal garden. Local climate conditions, such as temperature and rainfall, hold sway over the life cycle of these plants. Temperature affects everything from seed germination to flowering. A plant like rosemary, for instance, thrives in warm, sunny conditions, while others falter under the same intensity. Extreme temperatures can stress plants, leading to stunted growth or diminished potency. Rainfall, too, plays a critical role in influencing soil moisture levels and plant health. Herbs like lavender prefer well-drained, dry soils, but excessive rain can lead to root rot, compromising their vitality. Understanding these dynamics allows you to adapt your gardening practices, ensuring that your herbs reach their full potential despite the vagaries of weather.

Ginkgo Mocha Brain Latte

Brew ginkgo and ginger

Blend in 1 tsp cacao powder, ½ tsp lion's mane, a splash of oat milk, and a little vanilla

Sweeten with maple syrup

Frothy, rich, and perfect for creative focus

Adapting to climate challenges requires creativity and foresight. Utilizing microclimates within your garden can offer refuge for sensitive plants. These are small-scale climate variations created by structures, trees, or other features that provide shelter from wind or excessive sun. A wall that captures heat during the day and releases it at night can extend the growing season for warmth-loving plants like basil. Water conservation techniques are another key strategy. Drip irrigation systems deliver water directly to the plant roots, minimizing evaporation and ensuring efficient water use. Mulching helps retain soil moisture, reducing the need for frequent watering. These practices conserve resources and enhance plant health, fostering resilience in the face of climate fluctuations.

Selecting climate-specific plants that naturally thrive under your local conditions is a proactive way to mitigate climate-related challenges. In warmer climates, choose heat-tolerant herbs like oregano and thyme, which flourish under the sun and require minimal water. For regions with high rainfall, moisture-loving plants such as mint and comfrey can transform abundant water into lush, vigorous growth. These plants are well-adapted to their environments, offering reliable harvests with less intervention. By aligning your plant selections with the natural climate, you create a harmonious garden that thrives with minimal input, reducing stress on both plants and gardeners.

Oregano Pain Relief Wrap Recipe

Ingredients:

1 cup Fresh or ½ cup Dried Oregano Leaves – pain-relieving and warming
½ cup Dried Chamomile (optional) – calming and anti-inflammatory
1 tbsp Fresh or Ground Ginger – stimulates circulation and eases pain
1 tbsp Apple Cider Vinegar or Witch Hazel (optional) – reduces swelling
1 ½ cups Warm Water (not boiling, to preserve properties)
Soft Cotton Cloth, Cheesecloth, or Flannel Wrap

Instructions:

Make the Herbal Infusion:

Combine oregano, lavender, and ginger in a bowl or small pot.

Pour warm (not boiling) water over the herbs and let steep for 10–15 minutes.

Strain the liquid into a clean bowl, keeping the infused water.

Soak the Wrap:

Soak a warm herbal liquid in a cotton cloth, cheesecloth, or soft towel.

Wring out excess liquid so it is damp but not dripping.

Apply the Compress:

Place the warm wrap directly over the painful area (joints, lower back, neck, or abdomen).

Cover with a dry towel to keep the heat in.

Leave on for 15–20 minutes.

Reheat and repeat if needed.

Alternative Uses:

- ✔ *For Menstrual Cramps: Place on the lower abdomen for relief.*
- ✔ *For Joint Pain or Arthritis: Wrap around knees, elbows, or wrists.*
- ✔ *For Muscle Tension: Apply to the neck or shoulders.*

Boost the Effectiveness:

Add 2 drops of oregano essential oil (diluted in a carrier oil) before applying.

Alternate hot and cold wraps for circulation-boosting pain relief.

Pair with a gentle massage after using the wrap.

Proactive climate management means looking ahead and preparing your garden to withstand future changes. Installing shade cloths can protect delicate plants from the harsh midday sun, preventing leaf scorch and dehydration. Windbreaks, such as hedges or fences, shield plants from drying winds, conserving moisture and reducing stress. Diversifying your plant selections to include resilient varieties ensures your garden can adapt to shifting climates. This diversity creates a buffer against extreme weather events, as different plants respond uniquely to environmental stressors. By fostering a garden rich in variety, you cultivate resilience, safeguarding your herbal ecosystem against the uncertainties of climate change.

Creating a Self-Sufficient Herbal Ecosystem

Imagine your garden as a thriving ecosystem that sustains itself and supports your lifestyle with minimal external inputs. This vision of a self-sufficient garden becomes a reality when you reduce reliance on outside resources, creating a closed-loop system where each element complements and supports the others. In such a garden, the recycling of nutrients, water, and energy forms the backbone of sustainability. You become less dependent on store-bought fertilizers, pesticides, and even water as your garden evolves into an autonomous entity capable of nurturing itself and providing for your needs.

Implementing permaculture principles is a cornerstone of achieving self-sufficiency. Permaculture emphasizes using natural patterns and processes to design sustainable and efficient systems. By observing how nature operates, you can mimic these processes in your garden. For instance, incorporating diverse plant species encourages symbiotic relationships that enhance soil fertility and plant health. Companion planting and polycultures, where multiple plant types grow together, help maximize space and resources. The integration of animals, such as chickens or bees, can further support nutrient cycling and pollination, enriching the ecosystem. Composting is another vital technique, transforming kitchen scraps and garden waste into nutrient-rich compost that feeds your plants and improves soil structure. This closed-loop cycle reduces the need for synthetic fertilizers and enhances the resilience of your garden.

Natural Pesticide Spray for The Garden

This homemade herbal pesticide is safe, chemical-free, and highly effective against aphids, caterpillars, spider mites, whiteflies, and other common pests. It repels insects while protecting beneficial pollinators like bees and butterflies.

Why This Works:

✔ *Oregano & Garlic – Antimicrobial, repels pests, and prevents fungal diseases*

✔ *Neem Oil – Disrupts insect life cycles and acts as a natural insecticide*

✔ *Pepper & Vinegar – Deters bugs with its strong smell and taste*

✔ *Castile Soap – Breaks down pests' protective coatings and eggs*

✔ *Essential Oils – Extra repellent power (optional)*

Ingredients (Makes 1 Quart/1 Liter Spray):

2 tbsp Fresh or 1 tbsp Dried Oregano – Antimicrobial, repels insects

2 Cloves Garlic (crushed) – Repels aphids, caterpillars, and mites

1 tsp Cayenne Pepper or Red Chili Flakes – Deters chewing insects

1 tbsp Apple Cider Vinegar – Fungal prevention and pest deterrent

½ tsp Castile Soap (or mild dish soap, unscented) – Helps the spray stick to plants

1 tsp Neem Oil (optional but mighty) – Natural insecticide for severe infestations

3–5 drops Peppermint or Rosemary Essential Oil (optional) – Boosts pest-repelling power

1 Quart (4 cups) Filtered Water

Instructions:

Make the Herbal Infusion:

Bring 2 cups of water to a simmer.

Add oregano, Garlic, and cayenne pepper, then turn off the heat.

Cover and let steep for 30 minutes.

Strain & Cool:

Strain through cheesecloth or a fine mesh sieve.

Let it cool completely before adding other ingredients.

Mix the Spray:

Add apple cider vinegar, neem oil (if using), and Castile soap to the strained herbal liquid.

Stir well, then pour into a spray bottle.

Shake & Apply:

Shake before each use.

Spray directly onto plant leaves (top and underside) in the morning or evening.

Repeat every 3–5 days or after heavy rain.

Natural pest and disease management is pivotal in maintaining a healthy garden without synthetic interventions. Encouraging beneficial insects like ladybugs and lacewings provides natural pest control. These predators help keep harmful insect populations in check, reducing the need for chemical pesticides. Planting various flowering plants attracts these beneficial insects, creating a balanced ecosystem where pests and predators coexist. Herbal pest repellents, like neem oil or garlic spray, offer additional protection against pests without harming the environment. These effective and sustainable natural solutions ensure your garden remains safe for plants, animals, and people.

Integrating renewable resources into your garden further enhances its self-sufficiency. Rainwater harvesting systems, such as rain barrels or cisterns, collect and store rainwater for irrigation, reducing reliance on municipal water supplies. This practice conserves water and helps your garden withstand drought conditions. Solar-powered garden tools, like lights and pumps, harness renewable energy to minimize electricity consumption and carbon emissions. These tools provide a sustainable alternative to traditional, energy-intensive options, aligning your garden with eco-friendly practices. By utilizing renewable resources, you create a garden that sustains itself and contributes to the broader goal of environmental stewardship.

Soapy Water Spray for Roses

This gentle, natural soap spray protects roses from aphids, spider mites, and whiteflies while keeping their delicate leaves safe. It works by breaking down the outer coating of soft-bodied pests, effectively suffocating them without harming the plant.

Why Use Soapy Water?

✔ *Kills aphids, spider mites, whiteflies, and thrips*
✔ *Safe for beneficial insects when applied correctly*
✔ *Non-toxic and biodegradable*
✔ *Prevents powdery mildew and fungal growth*

Ingredients (Makes 1 Quart/1 Liter Spray):

1 tsp Liquid Castile Soap (or mild, unscented dish soap—avoid detergents!)
1 Quart (4 cups) Filtered Water

1 tsp Neem Oil (optional for more substantial pest control)

3–5 drops of Peppermint or Rosemary Essential Oil (optional, repels insects)

Instructions:

Mix the Ingredients:

Pour water into a spray bottle.

Add liquid Castile soap (or mild dish soap).

If using, add neem oil and essential oils.

Shake gently to mix.

Spray Application:

Spray directly onto affected leaves, stems, and buds (top and underside).

Apply in the morning or evening (avoid spraying in full sun).

Repeat every 3–5 days or until the pest problem is gone.

Pro Tips for Roses:

Test on a few leaves first to check for sensitivity.

Avoid spraying when temperatures rise above 85°F (29°C) to prevent leaf burn.

Rinse with plain water after 1–2 hours to prevent residue buildup.

Use weekly as a preventive measure during the growing season.

Mulch around roses with banana peels, eggshells, or compost for slow-release nutrients.

Trim off infected leaves to stop the spread of disease.

Improve airflow by pruning overcrowded branches.

Water at the base to avoid wet foliage, encouraging fungal growth.

As you cultivate a self-sufficient herbal ecosystem, you foster a deeper connection with the natural world. Each element of your garden works in harmony, creating a resilient and sustainable environment that supports your needs and those of the planet. This chapter has explored the principles and techniques for achieving self-sufficiency in your garden, setting the stage for a lifestyle that aligns with nature's rhythms. With these practices in place, your garden becomes a sanctuary of sustainability, a testament to the power of thoughtful design and ecological balance. In the next chapter, we will delve into building community and connection, exploring how your apothecary practices can foster relationships and inspire others to embrace a more sustainable way of living.

Chapter Nine
Building Community and Connection

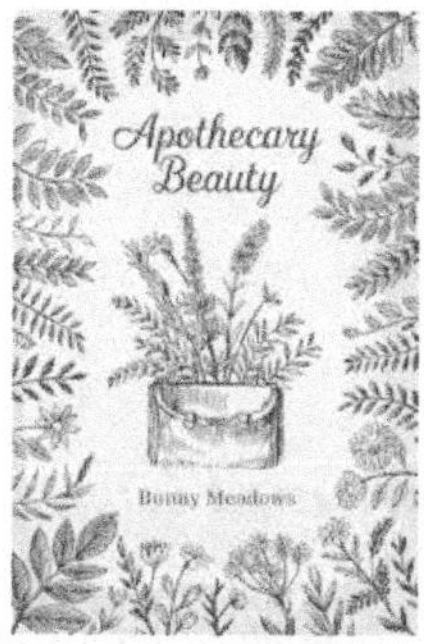

Imagine a garden as a vibrant tapestry of diverse plants, each one contributing its unique beauty and benefits. Now, envision this garden as a community of people, each bringing their knowledge and experiences to the collective. Just as plants thrive when they grow together, sharing nutrients and space, so do we benefit from the rich exchange of ideas and support in herbalist communities.

Finding and Joining Herbalist Communities

Connecting with herbalist communities offers immense benefits, providing a supportive network where you can deepen your understanding of herbal practices. In these groups, you gain access to shared resources and collective wisdom that can enhance your apothecary journey. Imagine being in a space where experienced herbalists share their tried-and-true remedies and cultivation tips, offering guidance that might take years to discover on your own. This access to knowledge accelerates your learning and empowers you to make informed decisions about your herbal practices. Moreover, the mentorship opportunities within these communities cannot be overstated. Experienced members often take newcomers under their wing, offering personalized advice and encouragement. Such relationships foster growth and confidence, allowing you to explore new facets of herbalism with the reassurance that seasoned guidance is available.

Fungal Prevention & Treatment Spray

This natural antifungal spray helps prevent black spots, powdery mildew, and rust, common rose diseases that thrive in humid conditions.

Ingredients (Makes 1 Quart/1 Liter):

1 tbsp Baking Soda – prevents fungal spores from spreading
1 tbsp Hydrogen Peroxide (3%) – disinfects and stops fungal growth
½ tsp Liquid Castile Soap – helps the mixture stick to leaves
1 Quart (4 cups) Water

Instructions:

Mix Water, baking soda, hydrogen peroxide, and Castile soap in a spray bottle.
Shake gently to combine.

How to Use:

Spray lightly on leaves, stems, and undersides every 7–10 days as prevention.
If fungal spots appear, apply every 3 days until improvement.
Do not spray in full sun—early morning or evening is best.
Protects from common fungal infections!

Finding the right herbalist community involves local and online exploration, each offering distinct advantages. Locally, herbal clubs and meetups are excellent starting points. These gatherings provide face-to-face interaction, allowing you to engage directly with others who share your passion. To find such groups, consider checking local community boards at libraries or garden centers or browsing event listings in newspapers and online platforms. Online communities offer another avenue, with forums and social media groups providing access to a global network of herbal enthusiasts. Websites like the American Herbalists Guild offer directories to locate herbalists and chapters in your area, making it easier to connect with nearby practitioners [Source 1]. Joining these online spaces allows you to exchange ideas and experiences with individuals from diverse backgrounds, enriching your understanding of herbalism on a global scale.

The diversity within herbalist communities is one of their greatest strengths, bringing together a wide array of perspectives and practices. You may encounter different cultural approaches to herbalism in these groups, each with unique traditions and uses. Some members focus on medicinal herbs, delving into plants' therapeutic properties and their healing applications. Others may be drawn to the culinary uses of herbs, creating vibrant dishes that celebrate flavor and health. Still, others explore herbalism's spiritual and ritualistic aspects, weaving plants into practices that connect them to the earth and their inner selves. This variety broadens your horizons, exposing you to new ideas and methodologies that can inform your practice.

Fertilizer Spray (Organic & Bloom-Boosting)

This homemade fertilizer provides essential potassium, nitrogen, and phosphorus for healthy blooms and lush foliage.

Ingredients (Makes 1 Gallon/4 Liters):

1 Banana Peel (chopped) – boosts potassium for intense blooms

1 tbsp Epsom Salt – enhances flower color and promotes magnesium absorption

2 tbsp Used Coffee Grounds (or 1 tbsp molasses) – adds nitrogen and beneficial microbes

1 tbsp Apple Cider Vinegar – balances soil pH for better nutrient absorption

1 Gallon of Water

Instructions:

Add banana peel, Epsom salt, coffee grounds, and apple cider vinegar to a large container with 1 gallon of Water.

Stir well and let sit overnight.

Strain (optional) and pour into a watering can or spray bottle.

How to Use:

Water roses at the base (not the leaves) every 2 weeks.

Use as a foliar spray (diluted 1:2 with Water) for extra nourishment.

It is best applied in the early morning or late afternoon.

Encourages lush foliage and vibrant blooms!

~

Engaging effectively with these communities involves active participation and a willingness to contribute. Volunteering at community events, such as herb walks or garden tours, provides opportunities to connect with others and learn hands-on. These events offer a platform to share your knowledge and experiences, fostering a spirit of collaboration and mutual learning. Whether you are a beginner or an experienced herbalist, sharing personal insights can spark discussions and inspire others. You contribute to the community's collective growth by offering your unique perspective. Engaging with these groups helps build relationships that extend beyond the meetings, creating a network of support and friendship that enriches your herbal journey.

Visual Element: Herbalist Community Resource List

Consider creating a resource list that includes local herbal clubs, online forums, and social media groups focused on herbalism. This list can serve as a valuable reference, helping you explore different communities and find those that align with your interests and values. Include contact information, meeting schedules, and key focus topics for each group.

The journey of finding and joining herbalist communities is deeply rewarding. It offers knowledge and support and a sense of belonging to a broader network of individuals who share your passion for plants and healing. Through these connections, you can cultivate a richer understanding of herbalism inspired by the diverse voices and practices that make up this vibrant community.

Hosting a Local Apothecary Workshop

Imagine inviting neighbors into your garden, the air filled with the scent of fresh herbs, as you share secrets of natural healing. Hosting a local apothecary workshop is a powerful way to foster community bonds and disseminate valuable knowledge. These gatherings create an opportunity to build regional networks, uniting individuals with a shared interest in herbalism. By offering a platform for education, you empower others to explore herbal practices, cultivating a community of informed individuals who can support one another. Workshops encourage open dialogue, where questions are welcomed, and experiences are shared, facilitating a collective learning environment. Participants leave with new insights and connections to like-minded individuals, strengthening the fabric of their local community.

Organizing a successful workshop begins with careful planning. Selecting an appropriate venue is crucial; whether it's your garden, a community center, or a local park, the space should comfortably accommodate all attendees and provide a suitable environment for planned activities. Consider factors such as accessibility, seating, and weather conditions if outdoors. Once you have a venue, setting a date that allows sufficient time for preparation and promotion is vital. An engaging workshop agenda is the backbone of the event, outlining the topics and activities that will captivate and educate participants. Consider incorporating a mix of presentations, demonstrations, and hands-on activities to cater to different learning styles. Gathering necessary materials and supplies is another critical step—ensure you have enough herbs, tools, and reference materials for all participants and any equipment needed for demonstrations.

Aloe Vera & Cucumber Hydration Cooler

A cooling, ultra-hydrating drink to soothe skin and reduce puffiness.

1 cup coconut water

½ cup fresh cucumber juice

1 tbsp aloe vera juice (pure, food-grade)

1 tsp honey

Ice cubes

To captivate your audience, choose topics and activities that resonate with their interests and needs. Hands-on herbal preparation sessions, where attendees can create their own tinctures or salves, offer practical skills they can take home and integrate into their daily lives. Plant identification walks can be informative and enjoyable, teaching participants to recognize and understand the plants in their local environment. Discussions on sustainable gardening practices can inspire participants to adopt eco-friendly methods in their gardens, promoting environmental stewardship alongside personal wellness. Tailoring the content to the interests of your community ensures engagement and participation, making the workshop a memorable and valuable experience for all involved.

Promoting your workshop effectively ensures a good turnout and maximizes its impact. Utilize social media platforms to reach a broader audience—create an event page, share enticing visuals, and post regular updates to generate excitement. Local bulletin boards at libraries, cafes, and community centers are also great places to advertise, reaching those who might not be active online. Collaborating with local businesses can expand your reach further; for instance, partnering with a health food store or nursery can provide mutual benefits through cross-promotion. These businesses may offer mailing lists or storefront space for flyers, helping you connect with potential attendees who share an interest in herbalism. By employing a multifaceted promotional strategy, you can ensure your workshop attracts a diverse and engaged group ready to explore the world of natural healing.

TCM Weight Management Tonic

This herbal tonic is inspired by Traditional Chinese Medicine principles. It supports metabolism, digestion, and balanced energy levels for natural weight management.

Ingredients:

Pu-erh Tea (Aged Black Tea) – 1 teaspoon loose leaf or one tea bag
Hawthorn Berries (Shan Zha) – 1 tablespoon dried
Ginger Root (Sheng Jiang) – 1-inch fresh, sliced
Cinnamon Stick (Rou Gui) – 1 small stick
Licorice Root (Gan Cao) – ½ teaspoon dried (optional for digestion support)
Raw Honey or Lemon – to taste (optional)
Filtered Water – 3 cups

Instructions:

Prepare Herbs: Rinse hawthorn berries and ginger slices lightly.

Simmer: Bring water to a gentle boil in a small pot, then reduce to a simmer. Add hawthorn berries, ginger, cinnamon, and licorice root. Let simmer for 10–15 minutes.

Steep Tea: Remove from heat, add Pu-erh tea, and steep for 5 minutes.

Strain & Serve: Strain the tonic into a cup. Add honey or lemon if desired.

Usage & Benefits:

Drink 1 cup in the morning and another in the afternoon to support digestion and metabolism.

- ✔ *Pu-erh tea aids in fat digestion and metabolism.*
- ✔ *Hawthorn berries promote healthy circulation and digestion.*
- ✔ *Ginger and cinnamon support warmth, digestion, and energy balance.*

Storage:

It is best enjoyed fresh, but can be stored in the refrigerator for up to 24 hours.

Support the body's natural rhythms with this gentle, metabolism-boosting tonic!

As you prepare to host your workshop, remember the importance of creating an inviting and inclusive atmosphere. Encourage participants to share their experiences and knowledge, fostering an environment where everyone feels valued and heard. This approach enriches the workshop and builds a sense of community, where each person's contribution enhances the collective understanding. Through these shared experiences, participants form bonds that extend beyond the event, creating a network of support and collaboration. Hosting a local apothecary workshop is more than an educational endeavor; it is an opportunity to cultivate community, inspire others, and contribute to a movement that values sustainability, wellness, and connection with nature.

Sharing Your Journey Through Digital Platforms

In today's interconnected world, the digital realm offers a unique opportunity to bridge the gap between distances, enabling herbalists to share knowledge and experiences across borders. Utilizing digital platforms connects you with a global audience and amplifies your voice, allowing you to reach others who are passionate about herbalism. By creating blog posts or vlogs, you can document your personal experiences and insights, transforming your journey into a resource for others. These digital diaries can capture everything from your successes and challenges in the garden to the nuances of crafting herbal remedies. Through social media, you can engage with audiences by sharing snapshots of your daily practices, fostering a sense of community among followers who appreciate the beauty and intricacy of herbal work.

Pineapple & Moringa Collagen Booster

Moringa is rich in vitamins A and E, which support collagen production and skin repair.

1 cup fresh pineapple juice

1 tsp moringa powder

1 tsp honey

Ice cubes

Selecting the right digital platforms is crucial for effectively reaching your desired audience. Instagram, for instance, is perfect for visual storytelling, allowing you to share captivating images of your garden, herbal creations, and the natural world. Its visually driven nature makes it easy to draw followers with stunning photos and concise captions.

On the other hand, YouTube is ideal for those who wish to provide more detailed tutorials and demonstrations, offering a space to delve deeply into topics like tincture-making or plant identification. This platform allows for longer-form content, where you can explain processes with clarity and depth, creating a library of educational videos that viewers can return to time and again.

Creating engaging content that resonates with your audience requires consistency and authenticity. Establish a regular posting schedule that keeps your followers engaged, whether weekly updates or monthly deep dives into specific topics. Authentic storytelling is key; sharing your genuine experiences, including the missteps, creates a relatable narrative that others can connect with. Transparency in your journey fosters trust, encouraging followers to engage with your content and share their own stories. Incorporating interactive content, such as Q&A sessions, invites your audience to participate actively, transforming passive viewing into a dynamic exchange of ideas. This engagement not only builds a loyal community but also enriches your own understanding through diverse interactions.

Nettle & Horsetail Hair Strength Tea

Rich in silica and minerals that support hair growth and strength.

1 cup hot water

1 tsp dried nettle leaves

½ tsp horsetail powder or dried horsetail

1 tsp honey

Optional: squeeze of lemon for flavor

Steep for 10 minutes, strain, and drink.

Collaboration with digital communities can further enhance your reach and impact. Partnering with other herbalists and creators for joint webinars or live streams allows you to combine audiences, providing a platform for shared learning and diverse perspectives. These collaborations can introduce you to new ideas and methods, broadening your horizons and deepening your expertise. Participating in digital challenges or campaigns can boost your visibility, aligning your content with trending topics and reaching audiences you might not have connected with otherwise. By engaging with these broader digital movements, you position yourself as an active member of the online herbalist community, contributing to and benefiting from the collective knowledge.

Digital platforms offer an expansive canvas to share your passion for herbalism, providing tools to connect, educate, and inspire. As you explore these virtual spaces, you'll find that they are not merely outlets for sharing information but vibrant communities where ideas flourish and connections are forged. Whether through a beautifully curated Instagram feed or an informative YouTube channel, your digital presence can become a beacon for those seeking guidance and camaraderie in their herbal journeys. Through these efforts, you contribute to a global dialogue on the power and potential of plants, enriching both your practice and the wider community.

Collaborating with Local Gardeners and Herbalists

Imagine stepping into a community garden bustling with activity, where the air is filled with the scents of fresh earth and aromatic herbs. In this vibrant setting, local collaboration becomes not just beneficial but transformative. Working alongside fellow gardeners and herbalists allows you to pool resources and share the workload, making seemingly daunting tasks more manageable. By exchanging seeds and plants, you expand the biodiversity of your garden and introduce new varieties that might otherwise be unavailable. Such exchanges also foster a sense of stewardship, as each participant becomes a custodian of the shared bounty, ensuring the preservation and propagation of diverse plant species.

Ingredients:

1 cup Medjool dates, pitted

½ cup almonds

½ cup cashews

¼ cup shredded unsweetened coconut

2 tbsp organic Ashwagandha powder

1 tbsp organic Shatavari powder

½ tsp cardamom powder

½ tsp cinnamon powder

Pinch of Himalayan pink salt

Additional shredded coconut or crushed pistachios (for rolling)

Directions:

Soak dates briefly in warm water; if firm, drain them.

In a food processor, blend almonds, cashews, coconut, Ashwagandha, Shatavari, cardamom, cinnamon, and salt into a fine crumble.

Add dates and blend until the mixture forms a sticky dough.

Roll dough into bite-sized balls.

Roll each ball in additional coconut or pistachios.

Benefits:

✔ Boosts vitality and energy

✔ Balances hormones and enhances mood

- ✔ Rich in antioxidants and adaptogens
- ✔ Supports digestion and overall wellness

Use: Enjoy as a nutritious dessert or energizing snack. Share generously!

Storage: Store refrigerated in an airtight container for up to two weeks.

To initiate these collaborations, consider attending local gardening events or markets. These gatherings provide a natural platform for meeting like-minded individuals who share your passion for herbalism. As you stroll through stalls brimming with produce and crafts, strike up conversations with vendors and fellow attendees. Expressing genuine interest in their work opens doors to future partnerships. Community garden projects also offer fertile ground for collaboration. Joining these initiatives allows you to contribute to a collective effort where everyone benefits from shared knowledge and labor. Whether building raised beds, planting communal crops, or organizing seasonal events, your involvement strengthens the community's ties.

Collaborative projects can take many forms, each offering unique benefits to the participants. Co-hosting community education events is one such example. By bringing together the expertise of multiple herbalists, you can offer workshops that cover a wider range of topics, appealing to a broader audience. These events can include demonstrations, talks, and interactive sessions, providing attendees with a hands-on experience that deepens their understanding of herbal practices. Group foraging excursions are another engaging activity. Gathering local plants in a group setting enhances safety and provides an opportunity to learn from each other's observations and techniques. These outings foster a deeper connection to the local environment as participants discover the natural resources available right in their backyard.

Nile Crocodile Wellness Cake Dessert

Nourishing & Delightful Ancient-Inspired Treat

Ingredients:

1½ cups almond flour (nutrient-rich base)

½ cup dates, pitted and finely chopped (natural sweetness)

¼ cup honey (energy and antioxidants)

3 eggs (protein-rich)

¼ cup coconut oil, melted (healthy fats)

1 tsp cinnamon (supports digestion)

½ tsp cardamom (warm, aromatic spice)

¼ tsp nutmeg (comforting flavor)

Optional topping: sliced almonds and drizzled honey

Instructions:

Preheat oven to 350°F (175°C); grease a cake pan.

Mix almond flour, dates, cinnamon, cardamom, and nutmeg in a bowl.

Whisk eggs, honey, and coconut oil in another bowl until smooth.

Combine wet and dry ingredients gently.

Pour into pan; bake 25-30 mins until golden.

Cool slightly; garnish with almonds and honey drizzle.

Benefits:

- ✔ Naturally energizing and nourishing
- ✔ Rich in nutrients and antioxidants

The benefits of collaborative learning extend beyond the immediate tasks at hand. Engaging with others allows you to gain insights into different gardening techniques, expanding your skill set and enhancing your apothecary practices. You might learn about innovative methods for pest control, soil enrichment, or water conservation that you hadn't considered before. Exposure to diverse herbal applications broadens your perspective as fellow practitioners share their experiences using herbs for culinary, medicinal, or spiritual purposes. This exchange of knowledge enriches your understanding and inspires creativity, encouraging you to experiment and innovate in your garden.

Learning is a reciprocal process in the community of local gardeners and herbalists. As you share your insights and experiences, you contribute to the group's collective wisdom. This dynamic interaction fosters a culture of mutual respect and appreciation, where everyone's knowledge is valued and celebrated. The relationships forged through collaboration are not just professional but often become personal, creating a network of support that extends beyond the garden. These connections offer encouragement during challenging times and celebrate successes, nurturing a sense of belonging and purpose. In this way, local collaboration becomes a cornerstone of your apothecary practice, enriching your journey with shared experiences and collective growth.

Building a Family Tradition of Herbalism

Incorporating family into herbal practices can transform the apothecary experience into something significant, fostering closer bonds and creating enduring memories. By inviting family members to participate, you open the door to shared learning and discovery. Teaching children about plant care and uses, for instance, educates them about the natural world and instills a sense of responsibility and curiosity. Imagine the joy of watching a child's eyes light up as they recognize a plant they've nurtured, understanding its potential to heal. These moments build confidence and create a foundation of knowledge that can be passed down through generations, ensuring that the wisdom of herbalism continues to flourish within the family.

Cinnamon Honey Lollipops for Wellness & Comfort

Delightful, warming cinnamon-infused lollipops, perfect for soothing sore throats, comforting coughs, and providing immune-boosting sweetness.

Ingredients:

1 cup raw honey (antibacterial and soothing)

¼ cup filtered water

1 ½ teaspoons ground cinnamon (warming and antimicrobial)

½ teaspoon vanilla extract (optional, enhances flavor)

Optional: pinch of ground ginger (extra warmth and anti-inflammatory)

Instructions:

Combine honey, water, cinnamon, vanilla, and optional ginger in a small saucepan.

Cook gently over medium-low heat, stirring continuously, until the mixture reaches 300°F (hard-crack stage) on a candy thermometer. (To test without a thermometer, drop a small amount into cold water—it should quickly harden and crack.)

Once at temperature, remove from heat and allow bubbles to settle.

Carefully pour into lollipop molds or onto parchment paper to form small discs; insert sticks immediately.

Let cool and harden completely at room temperature, then wrap individually in parchment paper.

How to Use:

Enjoy one lollipop whenever throat comfort or a warming treat is desired.

It is ideal during the cold season or for a comforting herbal sweet.

Benefits:

✔ *Throat-Soothing & Comforting – Honey and cinnamon calm sore throats.*

✔ *Warming & Immune-Boosting – Cinnamon enhances circulation and offers antimicrobial protection.*

✔ *Delicious, Natural Remedy – Perfect for adults and children.*

Family-friendly herbal activities provide an engaging way to involve everyone, regardless of age. Family gardening days can be an excellent opportunity to work together, transforming a patch of earth into a vibrant garden. This hands-on experience allows each member to contribute by planting seeds, watering plants, or pulling weeds. These activities teach patience and teamwork, as everyone shares in the labor and the rewards of a bountiful harvest. Crafting herbal remedies together, such as brewing teas or making salves, can be educational and fun. It's a chance to explore creativity while learning practical skills. As you measure and mix ingredients, conversations flow naturally, creating a space where stories of herbal traditions can be shared across generations. These stories, passed down, become a tapestry of family history, each layer adding depth and richness to the family's collective knowledge.

Passing on herbal wisdom to younger generations is vital to maintaining this tradition. Documenting family recipes and herbal lore is one way to ensure this knowledge is preserved. A well-worn notebook filled with handwritten notes and pressed leaves can become a treasured heirloom, a connection to the past. Involving kids in herbal preparation and gardening teaches them valuable skills and fosters a sense of pride and ownership in the family's herbal endeavors. They learn by doing, gaining firsthand experience that deepens their understanding and appreciation for the plants and their uses. This active participation helps to cement their connection to the tradition, encouraging them to carry it forward as they grow.

Herbal Gummy Bears for Immunity & Calm

These fun, colorful, and delicious herbal gummies are designed especially for kids to boost immunity, calm nerves, and encourage wellness.

Ingredients:

1 cup fruit juice (e.g., apple, grape, or cherry—preferably organic, no sugar added)

2 tablespoons raw honey or maple syrup (optional for sweetness)

2–3 tablespoons gelatin powder (grass-fed preferred, for gut and immune health)

Optional Herbal Boost (choose one or combine):

½ cup elderberry syrup (for immunity)

½ cup chamomile or lemon balm tea (for calming effects)

¼ teaspoon vitamin C powder (immune-boosting antioxidant)

Silicone gummy molds (bear shapes, hearts, stars)

Instructions:

Gently heat fruit juice, optional herbal tea or elderberry syrup, and honey/maple syrup in a small saucepan.

Sprinkle gelatin into the warm juice mixture, whisking continuously until fully dissolved, with no clumps (do not boil).

Remove from heat and carefully pour the liquid mixture into silicone molds.

Chill in the refrigerator for 1–2 hours or until fully set.

Pop gummies out and store them in an airtight container in the fridge.

How to Enjoy:

Kids can enjoy 1–3 gummies per day as a tasty wellness-boosting treat.

Benefits:

✔ *Boosts Immunity – Elderberry and vitamin C support immune health.*

✔ *Calming & Mood-Boosting – Chamomile or lemon balm gently soothes the nervous system.*

✔ *Supports Gut Health – Gelatin promotes gut lining repair and digestive wellness.*

✔ *Kid-Friendly & Fun – A playful and tasty way to introduce herbal wellness to kids.*

Creating lasting family traditions around herbalism involves establishing practices that resonate with the family's values and interests. A family herbal journal or scrapbook can serve as a living document, recording the family's herbal journey through photographs, drawings, and written reflections. This collective project encourages everyone to contribute, capturing milestones and discoveries along the way. Celebrating seasonal herbal festivals or events is another way to anchor these traditions in the rhythm of the year. Whether it's a midsummer harvest festival or a winter solstice tea party, these gatherings bring the family together to honor the cycles of nature and the fruits of their labor. These celebrations become cherished rituals, eagerly anticipated and fondly remembered, strengthening the family's bond and commitment to their herbal practices.

Through these practices, the family's connection to herbalism is woven into the fabric of daily life, enriching relationships and cultivating a shared sense of purpose. As each generation contributes to and learns from these traditions, a legacy is built that honors the past while nurturing the future. This chapter highlights the profound impact of involving family in herbal practices, emphasizing the joys and benefits of growing together in knowledge and experience. As you reflect on these ideas, consider how you might invite your own family into the world of herbalism, creating a tradition that will endure for years.

Chapter Ten
Beyond the Basics: Advanced Apothecary Techniques

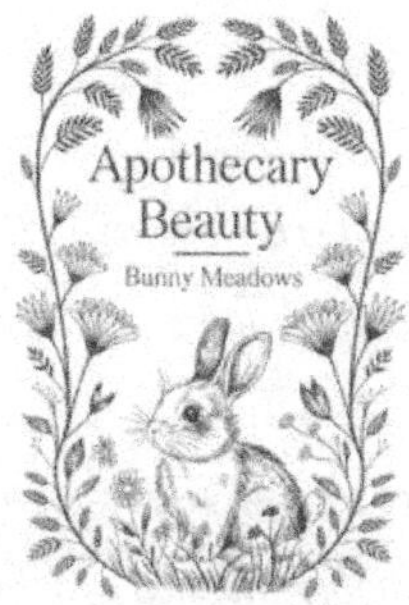

As the morning sun casts its golden light over your garden, each herb is a testament to nature's enduring wisdom. Advanced apothecary techniques invite you to deepen your practice, unlocking the full potential of these botanical allies. Picture yourself in your kitchen, surrounded by the vibrant colors and rich aromas of freshly harvested herbs. This chapter will guide you through the intricate art of creating tinctures, glycerites, and herbal vinegar, transforming your home apothecary into a sophisticated health and wellness hub.

Herbal Honey Tincture for Wellness & Immunity

A versatile, herbal-infused honey tincture that provides immune support, calming effects, and overall wellness benefits.

Ingredients:

1 cup raw honey (antimicrobial, soothing, and healing)
½ cup vodka or brandy (high-proof alcohol for extraction and preservation)

2 tablespoons dried herbs (choose one or combine: chamomile, lavender, lemon balm, elderberry, echinacea, thyme, or sage)

Optional: ½ teaspoon fresh lemon zest (immune-boosting and flavor-enhancing)

Instructions:

Place the dried herbs and optional lemon zest into a clean, dry glass jar.

Pour vodka or brandy over the herbs, ensuring they are fully submerged. Seal the jar and store it in a cool, dark place for 3–4 weeks, shaking gently every few days.

After infusion, strain out herbs using a fine-mesh strainer or cheesecloth.

Stir in raw honey until thoroughly blended.

Transfer to a clean glass bottle or jar and store in a cool, dark place or refrigerator.

How to Use:

Take ½ to 1 teaspoon directly or stir into herbal teas as needed.

Excellent for daily immune support, calming nerves, or soothing digestion.

Benefits:

✔ *Immune Support & Wellness Boosting – Herbal properties enhance overall vitality.*

✔ *Soothes & Calms – Perfect as a gentle relaxant or sleep aid (with calming herbs like lavender or chamomile).*

✔ *Digestive Comfort – Supports healthy digestion and gut health.*

✔ *Antimicrobial & Anti-inflammatory – Honey and herbs promote natural healing*

In herbalism, tinctures represent a powerful method for extracting active compounds from plants. Unlike basic infusions and decoctions, tinctures use alcohol as a solvent to draw out the therapeutic properties, resulting in a concentrated liquid that preserves the plant's essence. To create a tincture, begin by selecting high-quality alcohol, such as vodka or brandy. The proof of the alcohol is crucial, as it determines the extraction efficiency; 80 to 100 proof is generally recommended for most herbs. Measure your herbs carefully, typically using a ratio of 1 part herb to 5 parts alcohol for fresh herbs or 1:10 for dried. Combine the ingredients in a glass jar, ensuring the herbs are fully submerged. Seal the jar and store it in a cool, dark place, shaking it gently each day for four to six weeks. Once the tincture has matured, strain it through a fine mesh or cheesecloth to remove plant material, bottling the finished product in dark glass containers to preserve its potency.

Glycerites and herbal vinegar offer excellent alcohol-free alternatives, catering to different taste preferences and health considerations. Glycerites use vegetable glycerin, a sweet, syrupy liquid derived from plant oils, to extract herbal properties. They are particularly favored for their pleasant taste, making them ideal for children or those sensitive to alcohol. To make a glycerite, follow a similar process to tinctures but replace the alcohol with glycerin, maintaining the proper herb-to-solvent ratio. Herbal vinegars, on the other hand, utilize apple cider vinegar as the solvent, adding an acidic tang that enhances flavor and preservation. These preparations are perfect for culinary use, adding a zesty note to salads and dishes while delivering health benefits.

Herbal Sleep Tincture for Deep Rest

A gentle, effective herbal tincture carefully blended to encourage relaxation, ease stress, and promote restful sleep.

Ingredients:

2 tablespoons dried valerian root (deep relaxation and sleep support)
2 tablespoons dried chamomile flowers (soothing and calming)

1 tablespoon dried passionflower (relieves anxiety and promotes tranquility)

1 tablespoon dried lemon balm (mood-lifting and nerve-calming)

½ tablespoon dried lavender flowers (relaxing and sleep-inducing)

1 ½ cups vodka or brandy (high-proof alcohol for extraction)

Instructions:

Place all dried herbs in a clean glass jar.

Cover entirely with vodka or brandy, ensuring herbs are submerged.

Seal the jar tightly and store it in a cool, dark place for 4–6 weeks, shaking gently every few days.

After infusion, strain herbs using a fine mesh strainer or cheesecloth.

Pour tincture into an amber glass dropper bottle for easy use.

How to Use:

Adults: Take ½ to 1 teaspoon (approximately 20-40 drops) about 30 minutes before bedtime.

Dilute in a small glass of water or herbal tea for best results.

Benefits:

✔ *Promotes Deep, Restful Sleep – Valerian and Passionflower relax nerves deeply.*

✔ *Reduces Anxiety & Stress – Chamomile and lemon balm gently soothe the nervous system.*

✔ *Supports Relaxation & Calms the Mind – Lavender encourages tranquility and reduces mental chatter.*

Each extraction method brings its advantages, enhancing the versatility and longevity of your herbal preparations. Tinctures, with their robust extraction capabilities, offer the highest concentration of active compounds, ensuring maximum efficacy. Glycerites, while slightly less potent, provide a gentler alternative with a palatable sweetness. Herbal vinegars, meanwhile, offer a culinary twist, enriching your meals with both flavor and nutrition. Understanding these methods allows you to tailor your apothecary creations to suit your needs, preferences, and lifestyle.

Visual Element: Herbal Extraction Techniques Chart

Create a chart that outlines the steps, solvent options, and ideal ratios for tinctures, glycerites, and herbal vinegar. This visual aid will serve as a quick reference guide, simplifying the process and ensuring consistent results. Display it prominently in your kitchen or apothecary space for easy access, enhancing your confidence and efficiency in herbal extraction.

Proper storage and usage are essential to maintaining the quality and effectiveness of your extracts. Store tinctures, glycerites, and vinegar in dark glass bottles, away from direct sunlight and heat, to prevent degradation. Label each bottle with the herb name, extraction date, and dilution ratio, keeping an organized inventory. Use tinctures sparingly, as their concentrated nature requires only a few drops to achieve the desired effects. Glycerites and vinegar can be used more liberally, depending on taste and intended application. Adhering to these guidelines ensures that your advanced apothecary techniques yield potent, reliable remedies that enrich your health and well-being.

Crafting Herbal Elixirs, Syrups, and Tonics

Imagine your kitchen as a vibrant lab, brimming with the potential to craft elixirs, syrups, and tonics—each a unique blend of nature's gifts designed to support health and wellness. These preparations go beyond simple teas and infusions, offering a more complex approach to herbal remedies. Elixirs, typically alcohol-based, are potent brews crafted for specific conditions. They combine herbs to address targeted needs, such as boosting the immune system or enhancing relaxation. On the other hand, tonics are gentle, daily-use blends that sustain overall health. They incorporate herbs that support bodily functions and maintain balance. Syrups, with their sweet, viscous nature, serve as both medicine and delight, especially for those who may be averse to more pungent tastes. They are sugar-based, providing a palatable way to deliver herbal benefits.

Honey Throat Syrup for Soothing Relief

This gentle, soothing syrup, made with honey and herbs, is designed to calm coughs, soothe sore throats, and support respiratory wellness.

Ingredients:

1 cup raw honey (antibacterial and throat-coating)

¼ cup warm filtered water

2 tablespoons fresh lemon juice (vitamin C and detox support)

1 tablespoon fresh ginger, finely grated (anti-inflammatory and immune-boosting)

1 teaspoon cinnamon (soothing and antibacterial)

½ teaspoon turmeric powder (optional, reduces inflammation)

½ teaspoon thyme or sage (optional, respiratory support)

Instructions:

Gently warm (do not boil) the honey and water in a small saucepan over low heat, stirring until combined.

Stir in the lemon juice, ginger, cinnamon, turmeric, and herbs.

Let the mixture gently infuse on low heat for 5–10 minutes, then remove from heat.

Strain through a fine-mesh sieve into a clean jar, discarding solids.

Store syrup in the refrigerator for up to 3–4 weeks.

How to Use:

Adults: Take 1–2 teaspoons as needed, especially before bedtime or when experiencing throat discomfort.

Children (over age 1): Take ½ teaspoon as needed.

Benefits:

✔ *Soothes Sore Throats & Coughs – Honey and herbs coat and calm irritation.*

✔ *Boosts Immunity – Ginger, lemon, and turmeric support overall immune function.*

✔ *Reduces Inflammation & Supports Healing – Cinnamon and herbs offer antimicrobial properties.*

Creating herbal syrups begins by selecting a sweet foundation, such as honey or cane sugar, which acts as a preservative and a flavor enhancer. Start by simmering your herbs in water to extract their essence, then strain the liquid to remove plant materials. Return the decoction to the heat, gradually adding your sweetener, and stir until it dissolves completely. Continue to simmer until the mixture thickens to your desired consistency. Pour the syrup into sterilized bottles for storage. This process captures the herbs' therapeutic properties and balances sweetness with the medicinal flavors, resulting in a delightful concoction that can soothe a sore throat or boost immunity.

Herbal elixirs, meanwhile, require the art of maceration—allowing herbs to steep in a chosen spirit, often brandy or vodka, which acts as a solvent to extract and preserve their active compounds. Begin by selecting your herbs and chopping them finely to increase surface area. Place them in a glass jar, covering them entirely with your chosen spirit. Seal the jar and let it sit in a cool, dark place for several weeks, shaking it gently every few days. This process allows the flavors and medicinal properties to meld, creating a layered, rich elixir. Once ready, strain the mixture and store the elixir in dark glass bottles to protect it from light.

This method ensures potency and allows for the creative layering of flavors, such as combining cinnamon and anise for warmth or lemon balm for a citrusy note.

Elderberry Syrup

Immune-Supporting Herbal Syrup & Cake Garnish

Ingredients:

1 cup dried elderberries (or 2 cups fresh)
4 cups water
1 tsp cinnamon powder (or one stick)
½ tsp cloves (whole or ground)
1 tbsp fresh grated ginger
¾ to 1 cup raw honey (to taste)

Instructions:

Add elderberries, water, cinnamon, cloves, and ginger to a saucepan.
Bring to a boil, reduce heat, and simmer uncovered for 30–40 minutes.
Mash berries, then strain the mixture through a fine mesh or cheesecloth.
Allow to cool slightly, then stir in raw honey.
Pour into a sterilized glass jar or bottle. Store in refrigerator.

Usage:

Use as a cake drizzle or glaze
Spoon over warm desserts or pancakes
Stir into tea or warm water for wellness support.

Benefits:

- ✔ *Supports immune system*
- ✔ *Adds tart-sweet flavor to desserts*
- ✔ *Rich in antioxidants*

Consider crafting an immune-boosting elderberry elixir, combining elderberries with echinacea and a touch of ginger for warmth and spice. For an energy-enhancing adaptogenic tonic, blend ginseng with licorice root and a hint of cinnamon. These formulations provide synergistic effects, working together to amplify each herb's benefits. The balance of flavors and medicinal properties results in a harmonious blend that supports health while delighting the senses. Experiment with different herbs to tailor your elixirs to personal needs, adjusting adaptogen levels based on stress response or balancing warming and cooling herbs for holistic effects. Maintain a blending journal to record modifications, ensuring each creation is effective and pleasing to the palate.

Designing Personalized Herbal Blends

In the quiet sanctuary of your garden, surrounded by the vibrant hues and scents of blooming herbs, lies the potential to craft personalized herbal blends. These blends are explicitly tailored to meet your unique health goals, addressing personal concerns with precision and care. Whether you seek to enhance sleep quality, manage stress, or boost immunity, creating custom blends allows you to harness the nuanced properties of each plant. Imagine the satisfaction of sipping a soothing tea that you've meticulously crafted, knowing it's designed to ease your anxiety or lull you to sleep. This is the power of personalization in herbalism, where each blend reflects your needs and intentions.

When embarking on this creative process, it's important to understand the roles of different herbs. Begin by identifying primary herbs that directly target your health concerns. For instance, if you're crafting a blend for anxiety relief, chamomile and valerian root might serve as your primary herbs due to their calming properties. Next, incorporate supportive herbs that enhance the effects of your primary choices. In our anxiety blend, adding lemon balm and passionflower can provide synergistic support, creating a more potent remedy. Lastly, include synergistic herbs that bind the blend together, enhancing the overall harmony and effectiveness. These might be herbs like peppermint, which can improve the flavor profile and aid digestion, ensuring the blend is as enjoyable as it is effective.

Herbal Dry Shampoo (For Refresh + Volume)

Perfect for in-between wash days or scalp balancing

Base Powder Blend:

2 tbsp Arrowroot powder
1 tbsp Rhassoul clay or bentonite
1 tsp Finely powdered rosemary or lavender (dried and sifted)
1 tsp Cocoa powder (for darker hair tones)

Instructions:

Package in a shaker jar or paperboard sifter.
Optional: Add a few drops of lavender or rosemary essential oil and mix well.

Crafting these blends is both an art and a science, where intuition plays as crucial a role as knowledge. As you select and combine herbs, allow your insights and personal goals to guide you. Setting intentions for each blend can infuse the process with purpose, transforming it into a mindful practice. Are you seeking tranquility or vitality? Do you want to soothe body aches or uplift your spirits? By clearly defining your desired outcomes, you can align your choices to create blends that resonate deeply with your aspirations. As you work, trust your intuition to tell you when a blend feels right, whether it's the aroma, the taste, or how it makes you feel.

Consider some examples of personalized blends to inspire your creations. For a restful night's sleep, mix chamomile, valerian root, and lavender, known for their sedative qualities, with a hint of cinnamon for warmth. To ease anxiety, combine lemon balm, passionflower, and skullcap, herbs renowned for their calming effects. If stress relief is your goal, a blend of holy basil, ashwagandha, and peppermint can provide balance and rejuvenation. These examples offer a starting point, but remember, personalization is key. Adjust proportions and ingredients based on your experiences and preferences, allowing each blend to evolve as your needs change. Keep a journal documenting your experiments and results, noting what works best for you and refining your blends over time. This practice enhances your herbal knowledge and deepens your connection to the plants and their healing potential.

Innovating with Herbal Fermentation

Picture the bubbling effervescence of a homemade kombucha, alive with beneficial probiotics and rich in flavor, made right from the herbs you've nurtured in your garden. Herbal fermentation is an age-old technique that transforms simple herbs into dynamic, health-enhancing elixirs. This process not only enhances the bioavailability of the plant's nutrients but also introduces a complex and invigorating flavor. By fermenting herbs, you unlock their full potential, allowing beneficial microbes to break down plant fibers and making nutrients more accessible and easier for your body to absorb. This results in a drink or condiment that is delicious and packed with health benefits.

Basic Herbal Vinegar Formula with Variations

Ingredients:

Fresh or dried herbs of choice (see ideas below)

Raw, unfiltered apple cider vinegar (with "the mother")

Glass jar with a parchment-lined lid (vinegar can corrode metal)

Instructions:

Fill a clean jar about ¾ full with loosely packed fresh herbs or ½ full with dried herbs.

Pour vinegar over the herbs, covering them completely.

Cap tightly (line lid if metal) and label with herb and date.

Let infuse for 2–4 weeks, shaking gently every day or two.

Strain and store in a cool, dark place. Keep for 6–12 months.

Healing Herb Combinations:

Clarity & Brain Boost

Rosemary + sage + lemon peel

Great for salads, memory tonics, and early morning teas

Mineral-Rich Nourishment

Nettle + red clover + oatstraw

Add to broths, grains, or take by a spoonful daily

Digestive & Immune Tonic

Dandelion leaf + thyme + garlic + ginger

Use as a Fire Cider base or drizzle over roasted veg

Cooling & Calming

Tulsi + chamomile + lavender

Beautiful in a spritzer or bath vinegar

Heart & Skin Glow

Rose petals + hibiscus + lemon balm

Sweet, tart, and beautifying—great for face toners or mocktails

Why Herbal Vinegars?

Extract vitamins, minerals, and phytonutrients easily

Shelf-stable and long-lasting

Can be used internally (in food or as a daily tonic) or externally (as a hair rinse or toner)

Great alternative for alcohol-based tinctures—especially for kids or sensitive systems

One of the most rewarding fermented herbal products you can create is a ginger and turmeric kombucha. Start by brewing a black or green tea base, allowing it to cool before adding sugar and a kombucha starter culture, known as a SCOBY. As the tea ferments, fresh ginger and turmeric root are introduced and sliced thinly to infuse their vibrant flavors and potent anti-inflammatory properties into the brew. Allow this mixture to ferment for a week or two, tasting periodically until it reaches your preferred balance of sweetness and tang. Once complete, bottle your kombucha in airtight containers to carbonate, creating a fizzy, refreshing beverage that delights the palate and supports gut health with its probiotic content.

Fermented Herbal Honey

(a wild and sweet probiotic syrup)

Ingredients:

Raw honey

Fresh herbs (thyme, sage, holy basil, or rose petals work beautifully)

Optional: garlic or ginger for extra immune oomph

How-To:

Fill a clean jar ½ full with herbs.

Cover entirely with raw honey (stir to remove air bubbles).

Leave the lid slightly ajar, or use cheesecloth and a rubber band to let it breathe.

Stir daily for the first week.

After 2–3 weeks, strain or enjoy as-is.

Use in tea, on toast, or by the spoonful for a gut-friendly treat.

Herbal vinegar infusions offer another avenue for harnessing the potency of fermentation. Infuse apple cider vinegar with herbs like rosemary, thyme, or sage, allowing the mixture to steep for several weeks. The result is a robust, herbaceous vinegar perfect for culinary use, adding depth to salads, marinades, and sauces. The acidity of the vinegar acts as a natural preservative, capturing the essence of the herbs and ensuring a long shelf-life. Beyond its culinary applications, this infusion provides health benefits, including improved digestion and enhanced nutrient absorption.

Fermented Immunity Tonic (Fire Cider-Style)

This one is a potent probiotic. It is inspired by traditional fire cider but mellowed with herbs and fruit to balance the boldness. Perfect for adults!

Ingredients:

¼ cup Fresh Ginger Root (chopped) – anti-inflammatory

¼ cup Fresh Turmeric Root (chopped) – boosts immune response

2 tbsp Fresh Horseradish (optional but potent!) – clears sinuses and fights infection

4 Garlic Cloves (smashed) – antimicrobial powerhouse

1 tbsp Black Peppercorns – enhances turmeric absorption

½ Lemon (sliced, peel and all) – vitamin C

¼ cup Dried Elderberries – antiviral and immune-toning

1 tbsp Rosemary (fresh or dried) – antimicrobial and clarifying

2 tbsp Raw Honey – prebiotic, soothes the throat

2 cups Raw Apple Cider Vinegar (with the mother)

Instructions:

Use a mortar and pestle to mash ginger, turmeric, garlic, and peppercorns together.

Add all ingredients to a quart-size glass jar and pour vinegar until fully submerged.

Cover with a non-metal lid (or plastic wrap under the lid to prevent corrosion).

Store in a cool, dark place for 2–4 weeks, shaking daily.

After fermentation, strain and bottle the tonic. Add extra honey to taste if it is too spicy.

How to Use:

Take 1 tbsp daily for immune support.

During illness or exposure: 1 tbsp every 2–3 hours.

Add to tea, salad dressings, or dilute in warm water.

It tastes like a spicy-sour-sweet powerhouse tonic—warming and energizing!

Fermented herbs contribute significantly to gut health, a cornerstone of overall wellness. The probiotics produced during fermentation help balance gut flora, aiding digestion and boosting immunity. Regular consumption of fermented herbal beverages can improve digestive efficiency and enhance the body's ability to extract and utilize nutrients. However, to ensure successful fermentation, maintain a clean environment free from contaminants that could spoil your creations. Sterilize all equipment before use and closely monitor the fermentation process, watching for off-smells or mold that indicate contamination. With careful attention and practice, you can master herbal fermentation, transforming your garden's bounty into nourishing, flavorful concoctions that support health and vitality.

Integrating Modern Science with Traditional Practices

In herbalism, the fusion of modern science with traditional wisdom offers a powerful approach to health and wellness. This union validates ancient practices, bringing them into the contemporary spotlight with empirical research and scientific rigor. Traditional herbalism, once solely reliant on anecdotal evidence, now gains credibility through studies that reveal its efficacy. For example, turmeric, a staple in Ayurvedic medicine, has garnered attention for its anti-inflammatory properties. Clinical trials have demonstrated that curcumin, the active compound in turmeric, can rival synthetic drugs in reducing inflammation with fewer side effects. Such findings affirm traditional uses and expand the understanding of how these remedies work at a molecular level.

Applying scientific insights to traditional methods allows for refining and enhancing herbal practices. By adjusting preparation techniques, such as optimizing extraction methods or adjusting dosages based on new research, practitioners can increase the potency and efficacy of herbal remedies. For instance, recent studies suggest that pairing turmeric with piperine, found in black pepper, significantly enhances curcumin absorption in the body. This simple adjustment, grounded in scientific discovery, can transform a traditional practice into a more potent therapeutic tool. Embracing these advancements while maintaining respect for the origins of herbal knowledge enriches the practice and offers more robust health solutions.

Rhodiola Endurance & Recovery Elixir (For Athletes & Active People)

A muscle recovery and endurance-enhancing herbal elixir for athletes, fitness enthusiasts, or those recovering from physical exertion.

Ingredients:

½ tsp Rhodiola Powder – increases stamina and reduces fatigue
½ tsp Turmeric Powder – anti-inflammatory and muscle-soothing
½ tsp Ginger Powder – improves circulation and digestion
1 tsp Lemon Juice – detoxifies and adds vitamin C
½ tsp Raw Honey – replenishes energy
½ cup Coconut Water – hydrating and mineral-rich

Instructions:

Mix all ingredients in a glass of coconut water.
Stir well and drink before or after exercise.

Staying informed about the latest herbal research is crucial for anyone committed to effective apothecary practices. Engaging with academic journals and online databases dedicated to herbal medicine can provide valuable insights into emerging studies and breakthroughs. Websites like PubMed and herbal-focused publications offer access to a wealth of information covering everything from clinical trials to ethnobotanical research. Regularly consulting these resources helps you stay abreast of new developments, ensuring your herbal practices remain informed by the latest scientific knowledge. Additionally, attending conferences or joining professional associations can provide networking opportunities with researchers and other practitioners, further enriching your understanding and application of herbal science.

By balancing the wisdom of the past with the insights of the present, you cultivate an apothecary practice that is both rooted and innovative. This approach respects traditional knowledge while embracing the possibilities of modern science, offering a comprehensive view of herbalism that is both timeless and cutting-edge.

Foraging Wild Herbs Safely and Sustainably

Imagine setting off on a crisp morning, the forest floor soft beneath your boots, as you begin the rewarding practice of ethical wild foraging. This ancient art, grounded in respect for nature, requires a mindful approach. Sustainable foraging safeguards local ecosystems and honors Indigenous rights, recognizing many communities' deep cultural connections with the land. By foraging responsibly, you preserve biodiversity, ensuring these precious resources remain abundant for future generations.

To forage wild herbs effectively, equip yourself with knowledge and tools that enhance safety and success. Plant identification apps can be invaluable, offering instant access to databases that help confirm your finds and avoid dangerous lookalikes. These digital guides and a good field guidebook form a solid foundation for accurate identification, reducing the risk of harvesting incorrect or harmful plants. Be mindful of signs of overharvesting, such as sparse populations or visibly stressed plant communities, and move on if an area seems depleted. This awareness helps maintain ecological balance and ensures sustainability.

Brazil Nut & Reishi Adrenal Thyroid Tonic

Brazil nuts provide selenium, which is crucial for thyroid function, while reishi mushrooms support stress resilience.

1 cup warm oat or almond milk

2 crushed Brazil nuts (or ½ tsp Brazil nut powder)

½ tsp reishi mushroom powder

1 tsp honey

½ tsp cinnamon

Preparation and safety are paramount when venturing into the wild. Equip yourself with a well-stocked first-aid kit, ready to address minor injuries like cuts or scrapes that might occur. Dress appropriately for the terrain, wearing sturdy footwear and protective clothing to navigate through underbrush safely. Carry a small backpack with essentials, including water, snacks, and a compass or GPS device, to stay oriented and hydrated. Preparing for the unexpected enhances your foraging experience, allowing you to focus on the joy of discovery rather than potential risks.

The benefits of wild foraging extend beyond the physical harvest. It fosters a profound connection with nature, transforming each outing into a meditative experience. As you move through the landscape, you become attuned to the rhythms of the natural world, observing the interplay of plant and animal life that sustains these ecosystems. This connection nurtures a sense of stewardship, deepening your commitment to preserving these wild spaces. Yet, foraging also brings challenges, requiring patience and respect for the land. It calls for a keen eye, a willingness to learn, and an appreciation for the subtle cues nature provides. Through mindful foraging, you cultivate herbs and a greater understanding of your place within the natural world.

Future Trends in Home Apothecary

The landscape of home apothecary is undergoing a transformation driven by technological advancements and a growing desire for personalized wellness. One emerging trend is the increasing focus on tailored herbal medicine, where remedies are customized to meet the unique needs of individuals. This approach aligns with the modern emphasis on personalized healthcare, where one-size-fits-all solutions give way to treatments that consider personal health goals and genetic makeup. Imagine having an herbal remedy explicitly crafted for your stress levels or immune system, offering a bespoke approach to health that resonates on a deeper level.

Seaweed & Spirulina Thyroid Support Smoothie

Seaweed and spirulina are rich in iodine and iron, which are essential for thyroid health and hair strength.

1 cup coconut water

½ tsp spirulina powder

½ tsp kelp powder

½ banana

1 tsp chia seeds (for omega-3s)

Ice cubes

Innovations in herbal cultivation are reshaping how we grow and utilize plants. Hydroponics, a soil-free cultivation method, is gaining popularity for its efficiency and sustainability. By using nutrient-rich water solutions, hydroponics allows for precise control over growing conditions, leading to higher yields and faster growth cycles. This method is particularly beneficial for those with limited space or challenging climates, providing an accessible way to cultivate a diverse array of medicinal plants year-round. Coupled with this is the rise of digital tools for herbal education, enabling gardeners to deepen their knowledge and refine their practices. Apps and online platforms offer resources for identifying plants, tracking herbal intake, understanding the effects of various herbs, and fostering informed and empowered herbalists.

Herbal Hair Loss Shampoo

Herbal Hair Loss Shampoo

Root-nourishing • Scalp balancing • Hair-strengthening

Base Ingredients (Sulfate-Free Shampoo Base)

Use a clean, natural shampoo base:
½ cup liquid castile soap (unscented, gentle cleansing)
¼ cup aloe vera gel (soothes and hydrates the scalp)
2 tbsp vegetable glycerin (locks in moisture)
1 tbsp jojoba oil or argan oil (nourishes follicles without clogging pores)
1 tsp vitamin E oil (antioxidant and helps extend shelf life)

Herbal Infusion (Hair Loss Support):

Use as a strong tea and add to the shampoo base:
1 tsp rosemary – stimulates circulation and growth
1 tsp nettle – rich in iron and minerals
1 tsp horsetail – silica-rich, strengthens strands
1 tsp gotu kola – supports scalp circulation and collagen
1 tsp green tea – DHT blocker and antioxidant

Brew in 1 cup of hot water for 15–20 min. Strain, cool, and add to the shampoo base.

Essential Oils (Add ~20–30 drops total):

8 drops rosemary – energizes follicles
6 drops peppermint – stimulates growth, cooling
6 drops lavender – calming + soothing to scalp

4 drops cedarwood – balances oil production + DHT-blocking
2 drops tea tree (optional) – antimicrobial support
Instructions:
Mix the herbal infusion with the shampoo base

ingredients.
Add essential oils and stir gently.
Pour into an 8-oz dark glass with a pump or cap.
Shake before each use (natural separation is normal).
Massage into scalp, leave on for 1–3 minutes, then rinse.
Use 2–4 days a week for best results.

The role of technology in herbal practices extends beyond cultivation. Digital resources are enhancing how we learn, share, and engage with herbalism. Apps designed to track herbal intake and monitor effects allow users to document their experiences, providing valuable insights into what works best for their bodies. This data-driven approach supports informed decisions, helping individuals optimize their herbal regimens for maximum benefit. Additionally, online communities and forums connect herbalists worldwide, facilitating the exchange of ideas and experiences. These digital platforms offer a space for collaboration and support, bridging the gap between traditional wisdom and modern innovation.

Botanical Conditioner (Hydrating & Strengthening)

Detangles • Rebuilds strands • Soothes scalp.

Base:

½ cup natural conditioner base or unscented DIY blend (e.g., shea butter + aloe)

1 tbsp Aloe vera gel

1 tbsp Argan or Hemp seed oil

1 tbsp Herbal tea infusion (rosemary, horsetail, chamomile)

Optional Add-ins:

1 tsp Silk or oat protein (for shine and softness)

1 tsp Honey or glycerin (for moisture)

Essential oils: Lavender, Rosemary, Cedarwood (10–15 drops total)

How to Use:

Apply after shampooing, focusing on the ends. Leave in for 1–2 minutes, then rinse.

Embracing change and innovation in the apothecary world requires a balance of tradition and progress. While new technologies and methods offer exciting opportunities, it is vital to remain grounded in the time-tested principles of herbalism. Respect for traditional roots ensures that the wisdom of the past continues to guide us, even as we explore new frontiers. By integrating modern advancements with ancestral knowledge, we create a holistic practice that honors the integrity of herbal medicine while embracing its potential for growth and evolution. This open-minded approach invites curiosity and encourages a dynamic interaction with the natural world, enriching our understanding and appreciation of the plants that sustain us.

Conclusion

As we end our journey together in "The Apothecary Beauty Reset," I hope you feel empowered and inspired to embrace the transformative potential of home apothecary practices. Throughout these pages, we've explored the rich history and ancestral traditions of herbalism, reviving lost knowledge and integrating it with modern scientific insights. From understanding the basics of plant identification and cultivation to mastering advanced techniques like tincture-making and herbal fermentation, you now possess the tools to create a personalized apothecary that supports your unique health goals.

The path to holistic wellness is not just about the remedies you create; it's about fostering a deeper connection with nature and embracing a lifestyle that harmonizes with the earth. By practicing sustainable gardening, ethical foraging, and eco-friendly harvesting techniques, you become a steward of the environment, ensuring that the gifts of nature will continue to nourish and heal for generations to come. Remember, every seed you plant and every herb you tenderly nurture is a step towards a more balanced and vibrant future.

As you integrate these practices into your daily life, I encourage you to view this book as a starting point, a catalyst for further exploration and growth. Continue to deepen your knowledge through hands-on experience, seeking out workshops, foraging excursions, and connecting with like-minded individuals who share your passion for herbalism. The journey of a home apothecary is one of lifelong learning, where each season brings new insights and opportunities for discovery.

One of the most rewarding aspects of this path is the sense of community it fosters. By sharing your experiences, collaborating with others, and contributing to the collective wisdom of herbalism, you become part of a global network united by a common purpose. Whether you join local gardening clubs, participate in online forums, or host workshops in your backyard, engaging with this vibrant community will enrich your journey and provide endless inspiration.

As you embark on your transformative path, remember that lasting wellness extends beyond the physical realm. You cultivate a deeper connection to your body and spirit by crafting herbal remedies with intention and mindfulness. Each sip of a carefully blended tea or application of a lovingly crafted salve becomes an act of self-care, a moment to pause and reconnect with your inner wisdom. Embrace these rituals as opportunities to nurture not only your health but also your emotional and spiritual well-being.

So, my dear reader, I invite you to take the first step today. Start by planting a single seed, brewing a cup of herbal tea, or crafting a simple tincture. Allow these small acts to be the foundation upon which you build a lifelong practice of natural healing and self-discovery. Trust in the wisdom of the plants, the resilience of your own body, and the power of community to guide you on this transformative journey.

As I reflect on my path, I am filled with gratitude for the opportunity to share this knowledge with you. The wisdom contained within these pages is a testament to the countless generations of healers, gardeners, and nature lovers who have come before us, each leaving their mark on the tapestry of herbal tradition. By embracing these practices and making them your own, you become part of this rich lineage, carrying the torch of natural healing into the future.

Remember, the path of a home apothecary is not about perfection but progress. Embrace the challenges, learn from the setbacks, and celebrate the triumphs, knowing each step brings you closer to a life of balance, vitality, and connection. May the knowledge and inspiration found within these pages be a guiding light on your journey, illuminating the way to a more vibrant, health-conscious, and fulfilling life.

Stay curious, stay open, and stay connected. The world of herbal wonders awaits, and I am honored to have been a part of your journey. Until our paths cross again, may your gardens flourish, your remedies heal, and your spirit soar. With gratitude and blessings, your fellow apothecaries.

Acknowledgments

REFERENCES:

Iseum Sanctuary. (2020, April 2). *Magical herbal medicine of the ancient Egyptians.* Iseum Sanctuary. https://iseumsanctuary.com/2020/04/02/magical-herbal-medicine-of-the-ancient-egyptians/

Ventegodt, S. (2020). Comparison of the medical principles of the ancient Egyptian and the ancient Greek medicine, based on the medical papyri and *Corpus Hippocraticum. Journal of Alternative Medicine Research, 12*(2), 145-154.

National Center for Complementary and Integrative Health. (n.d.). *Ayurvedic medicine: In depth.* U.S. Department of Health & Human Services. Retrieved March 2, 2025, from https://www.nccih.nih.gov/health/ayurvedic-medicine-in-depth

Johns Hopkins Medicine. (n.d.). *Ayurveda.* Retrieved March 2, 2025, from https://www.hopkinsmedicine.org/health/wellness-and-prevention/ayurveda

Gonzalez, P., & Smith, R. (2020). *Celtic provenance in traditional herbal medicine.* National Library of Medicine. https://pmc.ncbi.nlm.nih.gov/articles/PMC7058801/

Field Mag. (n.d.). *A modern guide to ethical, sustainable foraging.* Retrieved March 2, 2025, from https://www.fieldmag.com/articles/sustainable-ethical-foraging-guide

Practical Self-Reliance. (n.d.). *16+ pollinator-friendly medicinal herbs.* Retrieved March 2, 2025, from https://practicalselfreliance.com/medicinal-herbs-plant-bees/

Roots and Refuge. (n.d.). *A complete guide to vertical gardening (on a budget!)* Retrieved March 2, 2025, from https://rootsandrefuge.com/vertical-gardening-on-a-budget/

Yale University. (n.d.). *The power of companion planting: A guide for your garden.* Retrieved March 2, 2025, from https://campuspress.yale.edu/wave/the-power-of-companion-planting-a-guide-for-your-garden/

Natural Resources Defense Council. (n.d.). *For thousands of years, Indigenous tribes have been planting for the future.* Retrieved March 2, 2025, from https://www.nrdc.org/stories/thousands-years-indigenous-tribes-have-been-planting-future

Smith, J. (2019). *Identification of medicinal plants by visual characteristics of leaves and flowers.* ResearchGate. https://www.researchgate.net/publication/337534280_Identification_of_Medicinal_Plants_by_Visual_Characteristics_of_Leaves_and_Flowers

Verywell Health. (n.d.). *10 healing herbs with medicinal benefits.* Retrieved March 2, 2025, from https://www.verywellhealth.com/healing-herbs-5180997

Mountain Rose Herbs. (n.d.). *How to make herbal infusions & decoctions for wellness.* Retrieved March 2, 2025, from https://blog.mountainroseherbs.com/herbal-infusions-and-decoctions

DIY Natural. (n.d.). *Make your own herbarium identification book.* Retrieved March 2, 2025, from https://diynatural.com/diy-herbarium/

Cleveland Clinic. (n.d.). *What are adaptogens & types.* Retrieved March 2, 2025, from https://my.clevelandclinic.org/health/drugs/22361-adaptogens

Singh, P. & Sharma, V. (2023). *Curcumin, inflammation, and neurological disorders. ScienceDirect.* https://www.sciencedirect.com/science/article/pii/S2213422023000471

McLean, W. (2020). Reviews of articles on medicinal herbs.

Australian Journal of Herbal and Naturopathic Medicine, 32(1), 32-36.

Murthy, M. N., & Shyamala, B. V. (2023). Human tau E14 mutation induced neurodegeneration in *Drosophila melanogaster* is ameliorated by developmental supplement of *Ashwagandha* root extract. *Journal of Complementary and Alternative Medical Research.* https://doi.org/10.9734/jocamr/2023/v22i3461

PubMed. (n.d.). *The effects of lavender and chamomile essential oil.* Retrieved March 2, 2025, from https://pubmed.ncbi.nlm.nih.gov/33454232/

Healthline. (n.d.). *12 science-backed benefits of peppermint tea and extracts.* Retrieved March 2, 2025, from https://www.healthline.com/nutrition/peppermint-tea

Mount Sinai. (n.d.). *Echinacea information.* Retrieved March 2, 2025, from https://www.mountsinai.org/health-library/herb/echinacea

Verywell Health. (n.d.). *Calendula: Uses, benefits, side effects, and more.* Retrieved March 2, 2025, from https://www.verywellhealth.com/health-benefits-of-calendula-4582641

World Health Organization. (n.d.). *Traditional medicine has a long history of contributing to conventional medicine and continues to hold promise.* Retrieved March 2, 2025, from https://www.who.int/news-room/feature-stories/detail/traditional-medicine-has-a-long-history-of-contributing-to-conventional-medicine-and-continues-to-hold-promise

Thank You for Joining the Apothecary Beauty Journey

You've reached the final pages of Apothecary Beauty, but your journey into natural healing and radiant well-being is just beginning. Through the wisdom of herbal remedies, time-honored beauty rituals, and the power of a home apothecary, we hope this book has inspired you to embrace a more holistic and self-sufficient approach to health and beauty.

We'd Love to Hear From You

Your thoughts and experiences are invaluable—not just to us, but to fellow readers who are curious about the world of natural beauty. Did a particular recipe or remedy make a difference in your routine? Were you surprised by the simplicity and effectiveness of botanical skincare? How has this book changed the way you approach self-care?

Leave a Review - Whether on a bookseller's website, social media, or a personal blog, your words help others discover the magic of natural beauty and holistic healing.

Keep the Magic Alive

The journey doesn't end here. Continue experimenting, crafting, and deepening your connection to nature's remedies. Join our community of like-minded herbal enthusiasts, share your own discoveries, and keep embracing the beauty of a home apothecary.

Thank you for being part of this journey. Your voice helps keep the wisdom of herbal beauty alive for generations to come.

Made in the USA
Monee, IL
13 September 2026

63137527R00134